The All-in-One Guide to Herbs, Vitamins & Minerals

Victoria Hogan

Published by *alive* books
7436 Fraser Park Drive
Burnaby BC Canada V5J 5B9
(604) 435-1919 or (800) 663-6580

Copyright 1996

Cover Design: Peter Virag
Layout & Type Design: Irene Hannestad
Colour Photographs: Siegfried Gursche
                    Except where otherwise credited

First Printing - August 1996
Second Printing - September 1997
Third Printing - May 1999
Fourth Printing - August 1999

Canadian Cataloguing in Publication Data
Hogan, Victoria, 1957-
   The all-in-one guide to herbs, vitamins and minerals

   Includes index.
   ISBN 0-920470-99-8

   1. Herbs--Therapeutic use--Handbooks, manuals, etc. 2.
   Vitamins--Handbooks, manuals, etc. 3. Vitamin therapy--
   Handbooks, manuals, etc. I. Title.
   RM666.H33H63 1996   615'.321   C96-910520-7

Printed and bound in Canada

Table of Contents

Introduction

Congratulations! Reading this book is the first step toward taking charge of your health. Herbs, vitamins and minerals have been around for humankind's history, and ancient people knew what to do with them to heal themselves and gain optimal health. They also knew instinctively what foods to eat in order to stay healthy without knowing the names of the individual vitamins and minerals contained in those foods.

But, modern post-industrial life has put a lot of unhealthy and dangerous substances into our air, food and water. Farmers used to raise wholesome foods, but the agriculture business now uses an array of toxic chemicals and, because of this and overdevelopment, the once-rich soils of this continent have been depleted. Processed foods do not give us the natural balance of nutrients our grandparents enjoyed. So now, with cutbacks in spending on medical services, it is up to each individual to find ways to, first of all, stay healthy, and secondly, find remedies for many of the ailments that have become more frequent in our stressful, hectic lives.

Modern medicine has turned its back on traditional ways, depending more on pharmaceutical drugs and sophisticated medical treatments. However, more and more medical doctors are realizing that vitamins, minerals and herbs have a place in the healing process. While in most European and Asian countries health care providers and individuals have long recognized the value of natural healing techniques, North America is only now taking notice. Famous Western doctors are writing books on the benefits of preventive and natural medicine. For example, Dr. Andrew Weil, a Harvard MD, now teaches a credit course in alternative medicine at the University of Arizona medical school. Talk with your health care provider and show him or her this guide. Many doctors are now open to discussing and using these time-proven methods.

This guide will help you make informed choices on the many herb, vitamin and mineral products available today. Remember that each person is unique, biochemically, genetically and environmentally, so what may work for one person may not be right for another. Experiment with dosages, notice the effects and adjust accordingly. As with any health care program, it is a good idea to work with your doctor or naturopath, follow product label instructions carefully and be cautious when administering to young children and pregnant women. Good luck and enjoy the rewards of ideal health, the natural way!

Part 1

Vitamins and Minerals

*M*ost people think of vitamins as pills, to be used like drugs. This could not be farther from the truth. Vitamins are organic substances required for life, essential to the normal functioning of our bodies and necessary for growth, vitality and well-being. All organic foods contain minute amounts of vitamins and minerals, but many of our manufactured foods, and even products, grown on depleted soils may lack adequate vitamins and minerals.

Vitamins work synergistically. This means vitamins work together with other vitamins to maximize their effectiveness, so it is important to have a balance. Experts have given us the Recommended Daily Allowances, or the RDA, but these may vary for individuals and circumstances. For example, smokers and older people, as well as people working or living in more toxic conditions, may have a higher need for some vitamins. To get around these variations, the experts add in a Margin of Allowance, which means they recommend 5, 10 or up to 1,000 times more than the RDA. Avoid confusion by using common sense. By knowledgeably experimenting with dos-ages and noticing the effects, you can come to a dosage that is right for you.

Antioxidants are important to modern life to combat free radicals. In the environment and in our bodies molecular by-products are created called free radicals. Free radicals are molecules with an unpaired electron that steal electrons from other molecules. These highly reactive particles can cause oxidative or oxygen-burning damage which has been linked to cancer, heart disease, arthritis, cataracts and even the aging process.

The body has a system of antioxidants or enzymes and nutrients that protects it from oxidative cell damage. When there is a good supply of antioxidants, free radical damage is held in check. Vitamins A, C and E, and the minerals selenium and zinc are common and effective antioxidants.

Though all vitamins and minerals are available in foods, given the denatured and processed foods available, the only sure way to know we are getting healthy amounts of all these nutrients is by taking supplements.

2 Vitamins and Minerals

Supplementing our diet with vitamins and minerals saves us time and worry, and assures us that we are doing our part to keep ourselves and our families in robust health. Remember that all doctors, naturopaths and herbalists first recommend eating a natural whole foods diet and exercising regularly to form a solid foundation on which to build good health.

Although most vitamin and mineral guides have traditionally listed best sources for certain vitamins and minerals as liver and fish liver oils, the consumer should be aware that the liver is the organ which handles toxic substances in an animal's body. Being responsible for processing the residue of our polluted environment and excessive use of chemicals, plus all the runoff into our streams, rivers and oceans of mercury, PCBs and other toxic substances, makes liver a potentially risky choice when supplementing for good health. Milk products and eggs have similar risks, as bio-accumulating pesticides, hormones, antibiotics and chemicals wind up in the fat of animals who ingest them. If you choose to use dairy products and eggs, you will optimize your health by using organically raised products. Furthermore, only animal products, not plant products, contain cholesterol. Many of North America's most serious diseases, such as heart disease, certain types of cancers, diabetes and kidney disease, are linked to the typical Western high-fat, high-protein diet. For this reason, an ideal diet is predominantly plant-based and includes the Recommended Daily Allowances of vitamins and minerals.

The vitamins in this guide are designated as either water or fat soluble. Vitamins A, D and E are fat soluble, and need some fat for proper assimilation. This means it is best to take these with some food that contain fat, such as a few almonds, sunflower seeds, peanuts or peanut butter, or with a meal, since meals contain some fat content. Fat soluble vitamins may be stored in the body, unlike water soluble vitamins which need to be replenished on a daily basis. Some water soluble vitamins, such as C, should be taken throughout the day in smaller doses for optimum protection and effectiveness. One large dose of water soluble vitamins may be wasted, as they are quickly absorbed, and any excess isexcreted in the urine in two or three hours. To avoid taking supplements all day, there are now time-released capsules. For anyone on a fat-restriced diet, there are dry forms of vitamins A, D and E available which are not fat-based.

Vitamins should be stored in a cool dark place, and kept away from sunlight to preserve the shelf-life of the products. Most vitamins have expiry dates, but this may vary slightly, depending on storage conditions. Most vitamins and minerals will last two or three years if kept in a proper container under optimal conditions. The best time to take vitamins is shortly after a meal, and preferably after each meal throughout the day. If this is too complicated, take them twice a day, after breakfast before leaving home, and again after the evening meal. Otherwise, take all your supplements after your biggest meal, usually in the evening.

Guide to Vitamins

Vitamin A

(Fat Soluble) RDA 5000 IU
Should be taken with food, preferably with fat or oil. Can be stored in the body, so not needed daily. Two forms: Retinol, found only in animal foods, and carotene, both plant and animal origin.

What It Does: Produces visual purple for night vision and maintains eyesight. Builds resistance to infection and healthy bones, teeth, skin, hair and gums. Helps delay senility and prolong longevity.

Health Benefits: Helps acne, alcoholism, allergies, arthritis, asthma, athlete's foot, boils, bronchitis, colds, cystitis, diabetes, eczema, heart disease, migraine headaches, hyperthyroidism, psoriasis, sinusitis, stress, loss of smell, poor appetite, tooth and gum disease, fatigue and loss of energy.

Sources: Fish liver oils, dairy products, tomatoes and all green and yellow fruits and vegetables.

Friends: B-complex, choline, vitamins C, D and E, calcium, phosphorous and zinc.

Enemies: Polyunsaturated fatty acids with carotene need antioxidants present or vitamin A becomes ineffective.

Cautions: Do not exceed 50,000 IU daily in adults for several months, or 18,500 IU daily for children.

Vitamin B1

(Thiamine) (Water Soluble) RDA 1.4 mg
Not stored in the body, so should be taken daily. Needs increase during stress, illness or surgery.

What It Does: Promotes appetite, builds blood, aids carbohydrate metabolism, circulation, digestion, energy, growth and learning capacity. Prevents water retention, constipation and helps fight motion sickness.

Health Benefits: Helps alcoholism, anemia, fluid retention, constipation, diarrhea, diabetes, indigestion, lead poisoning, nausea, mental illness, pain, rapid heart rate and stress.

Sources: Nutritional yeast, whole wheat, oatmeal, peanuts, rice husks, seeds, nuts, soy beans, most vegetables and dairy products.

Friends: B-complex, B2, folic acid, niacin, vitamins C and E, and manganese. B1, B2 and B6 should be equally balanced.
Enemies: Heat from cooking destroys vitamin B1 as does caffeine, alcohol, food processing methods, air, water, estrogen and sulfa drugs.

Cautions: No known toxicity. Excess is excreted in the urine and not stored in the tissues.

Vitamin B2

(Riboflavin) (Water Soluble) RDA 1.6 mg
Not stored in the body, so should be taken daily. Increased need during stress, pregnancy and lactation. North America's most common vitamin deficiency.

What It Does: Aids growth, reproduction and is involved in breakdown and use of protein, fats and carbohydrates. Promotes healthy skin, nails and hair, and helps vision and eye fatigue.

Health Benefits: Helps arteriosclerosis, high cholesterol, cystitis, hypoglycemia, light sensitivity, muscular disorders, nervous disorders, nausea in pregnancy, dizziness and baldness.

Sources: Milk, liver, cheese, fish, eggs, whole grains, nutritional yeast, wheat germ, leafy green vegetables, almonds and sunflower seeds.

Friends: B-complex, B3, B6 and C.

Enemies: Sunlight, alkalies, water (B2 dissolves in cooking liquids), alcohol, estrogen and sulfa drugs.

Cautions: No known toxic effects.

Vitamin B3

(Niacin)(Water Soluble) RDA 20 mg
The body can make its own niacin using the amino acid tryptophan, unless B1, B2 and B6 are deficient. Niacin causes flushing, but the niacinamide form does not have this effect.

What It Does: Used to breakdown and utilize proteins, fats and carbohydrates. Improves circulation, reduces cholesterol, maintains healthy skin, tongue and digestive tissues, and is needed for nervous system function.

Health Benefits: Helps acne, diarrhea, alcoholism, headaches, indigestion, insomnia, depression, fatigue, muscular weakness, nausea and high cholesterol.

Sources: Liver, lean meat, whole wheat products, nutritional yeast, fish, eggs, white meat of poultry, avocados, dates, fits and prunes.

Friends: B-complex, B5, B12, biotin, and vitamin C.

Enemies: Food processing methods, water, alcohol, estrogen, sleeping pills and sulfa drugs.

Cautions: Nontoxic, but doses above 100 mg may cause flushing.

Vitamin B5

(Pantothenic Acid) (Water Soluble) RDA 10 mg
Can be synthesized in the body by intestinal bacteria. A stress vitamin, so take extra during stressful times.

What It Does: Helps to convert fat and sugar into energy and is vital for function of adrenal glands. Helps in cell building, and maintenance of the central nervous system, and keeps skin and intestines healthy.

Health Benefits: Helps high cholesterol, allergies, asthma, arthritis, baldness, cystitis, digestive problems, duodenal ulcers, hypoglycemia, tooth decay and stress.

Sources: Nutritional yeast, whole grains, green vegetables, nuts, meat and unrefined molasses.

Friends: B-complex, B6, B12, biotin, folic acid and vitamin C.

Enemies: Heat, food processing, caffeine, estrogen, alcohol, sleeping pills and sulfa drugs.

Cautions: Nontoxic

Vitamin B6

(Pyridoxine) (Water Soluble) RDA 2 mg
Replace daily with foods or supplement. Take more with high protein diet and with pregnancy, lactation or if taking the birth control pill. Needed for producing antibodies and red blood cells.

What It Does: Used to assimilate proteins, fats and vitamin B12. Helps maintain the balance between sodium and potassium, which promotes normal function of the nervous and musculo-skeletal systems.

Health Benefits: Helps acne, anemia, arthritis, depression, dizziness, nervous disorders, hair loss, irritability, learning disabilities and muscle spasms.

Sources: Nutritional yeast, wheat germ, mushrooms, nuts, liver, broccoli, asparagus, lima beans, lettuce, spinach and dark green leafy vegetables.

Friends: B-complex, B1, B2, B5, C, magnesium and potassium.

Enemies: Food processing techniques, long storage, water, alcohol and estrogen.

Cautions: Nontoxic, but supplementing more than 200mg per day may result in vivid dream recall and night restlessness.

Biotin

(one of B-complex) (Water Soluble) RDA 3 mcg
Can be synthesized by intestinal bacteria. Usually measured in micrograms. Needed for synthesizing ascorbic acid.

What It Does: Helps keep hair from turning gray and prevents baldness. Alleviates eczema and dermatitis.

Health Benefits: Helps some skin conditions, eczema, hair loss, depression, fatigue, insomnia, muscular pain and poor appetite.

Sources: Nuts, fruits, nutritional yeast, egg yolk, milk and unpolished rice.

Friends: B-complex, B5, B12, folic acid and vitamin C.

Enemies: Raw egg white prevents absorption by the body. Water, estrogen, food processing, alcohol and sulfa drugs.

Cautions: Nontoxic

Choline

(B-complex) (Water Soluble) RDA N/A
This fat emulsifier or lipotropic works with inositol to use fats and cholesterol in the body. Maximizes effectiveness of vitamin E. Can penetrate the "blood-brain barrier", or the barrier that protects the brain from differences in diet that affect the blood, and helps produce a chemical involved in memory.

What It Does: Helps control cholesterol and send nerve impulses to the brain. Aids liver in eliminating poisons and drugs from the system.

Health Benefits: Reduces cholesterol and prevents colds, with A and C. Helps alcoholism, anemia, arteriosclerosis, cirrhosis, diarrhea, fatigue, menstrual problems, mental illness, ulcers and stress.

Sources: Egg yolks, green leafy vegetables, nutritional yeast, wheat germ, lecithin and liver.

Friends: Vitamin A, B-complex, B12, folic acid and inositol.

Enemies: Food processing, estrogen, alcohol, water and sulfa drugs.

Cautions: Nontoxic

Folic Acid
(B-complex) (Water Soluble) RDA 400 mcg
Essential for forming red blood cells, division of body cells, helps protein assimilation and production of nucleic acids (RNA and DNA). Pregnant women need double recommended dose.

What It Does: Improves lactation, protects against intestinal parasites and food poisoning. Relieves pain, improves appetite, helps circulation and skin conditions, fatigue, mental depression and graying hair.

Health Benefits: Helps anemia, arteriosclerosis, baldness, high cholesterol, constipation, heart disease, weight problems and loss of libido.

Sources: Nutritional yeast, wheat germ, mushrooms, nuts, broccoli, dark green vegetables and liver.

Friends: B-complex, B5, B12, biotin, and vitamin C.

Enemies: Food processing, heat, water, sunlight, estrogen and sulfa drugs.

Cautions: Nontoxic, but a few experience skin reactions.

Inositol
(B-complex) (Water Soluble) RDA 250 - 500 mcg
Important in nourishing brain cells. Heavy coffee drinkers probably need to supplement. Maximizes effectiveness of vitamin E.

What It Does: Helps lower cholesterol levels and metabolize and redistribute fats. Promotes healthy hair, prevents thinning and baldness, helps prevent eczema and helps brain cells by metabolizing lecithin.

Health Benefits: Helps alcoholism, anemia, arteriosclerosis, baldness, cirrhosis, diarrhea, fatigue, menstrual problems, mental illness, stomach ulcers and stress.

Sources: Nutritional yeast, dried lima beans, cantaloupe, grapefruit, raisins, wheat germ, unrefined molasses, peanuts, cabbage and liver.

Friends: B-complex, B12 and choline.

Enemies: Food processing, water, alcohol, coffee, estrogen and sulfa drugs.

Cautions: Nontoxic

PABA
(B-complex) (Water Soluble) RDA N/A
Known for its sunscreening properties. May help, with pantothenic acid to restore gray hair. Important in processing protein.

What It Does: Important for cellular metabolism. Helps maintain a healthy digestive tract. Stimulates adrenal glands and is important to healthy skin and nerves.

Health Benefits: Helps muscle cramps, gastro-intestinal disturbances, stress and infertility. Protects against sunburn, keeps skin healthy and smooth, may help restore natural color to gray hair.

Sources: Nutritional yeast, molasses, rice bran, whole grains, green vegetables, peas, beans, peanuts, egg yolk and liver.

Friends: B-complex, folic acid and vitamin C.

Enemies: Food processing, water, alcohol, estrogen and sulfa drugs.

Cautions: Nontoxic, but do not take high doses for long time. Nausea or vomiting may indicate an excessive dosage.

Vitamin B12

(Water Soluble) RDA 6 mcg
Produced in the stomach by the friendly bacteria often found on organic vegetables. Mistakenly thought to be only found in animal products. Can be stored in body for five years or longer. Known as cobalamin, it should be combined with calcium to absorb properly. Needed in very small amounts, but should be supplemented if on vegan (pure vegetarian) diet, though microscopic bacteria on organic vegetables can often help supply the requirement.

What It Does: Needed for metabolism of nerve tissue. Helps in protein, fat and carbohydrate metabolism. Forms and regenerates red blood cells, thus preventing anemia. Improves energy, appetite, concentration, memory and balance.

Health Benefits: Helps fatigue, anemia, baldness, eczema and leg cramps.

Sources: Sea vegetables such as kombu, hijiki, arame, wakane and black nori, blue-green algae, chlorella, barley green and spirulina, meats and dairy products.

Friends: B-complex, B6, C, choline, folic acid, inositoland potassium.

Enemies: Sunlight, water, acids and alkalies, alcohol, estrogen and sleeping pills.

Cautions: Nontoxic, even with megadoses, as some doctors give B12 shots.

Vitamin B13

(Orotic Acid) RDA N/A
What It Does: May help prevent premature aging and some liver problems.

Health Benefits: Helps multiple sclerosis.

Sources: Root vegetables and whey.

Friends: B-complex

Enemies: Water and sunlight.

Cautions: More research is necessary. Best to use with advice of health care practitioner.

Vitamin B15

(Pangamic Acid) (Water Soluble) RDA N/A, but 100 mg suggested
Not a vitamin in the strict sense, as essential requirement not proven,

but good results have been found, especially in Russia.

What It Does: Extends cell life span, stops craving for alcohol, helps fatigue recovery, lowers cholesterol, protects against pollutants, protects from cirrhosis of liver and stimulates immune system.

Health Benefits: Helps hangovers, glandular and nerve problems, heart disease, diminished oxygen to tissues and handling of heavy pollution.

Sources: Nutritional yeast, brown rice, whole grains, pumpkin and sesame seeds.

Friends: Vitamins A and E.

Enemies: Water and sunlight.

Cautions: More research necessary, but no toxicity known. Some have nausea at first, but if taken after a large meal, this should not be a problem.

Vitamin B17
(Laetrile) RDA N/A
A controversial "vitamin" used as an alternative aid to help cancer sufferers.

What It Does: Has the reputation of helping to prevent cancer.

Health Benefits: Helps prevent and heal cancer, by anecdotal reputation.

Sources: Apricot pits, apples, plums and peaches.

Friends: Unknown

Enemies: Unknown

Cautions: Because apricot pits contain cyanide, taking large amounts may be dangerous. Not more than 1 gram at any one time, and cumulatively, not more than 3 grams.

Vitamin C
(Ascorbic Acid) (Water Soluble) RDA 60 mg
Probably the most popular vitamin. Humans must rely on dietary sources. Used up faster under stress. The elderly and smokers have higher needs (each cigarette destroys 25 mg). Best to take time-released supplement to maintain high dose, as it is excreted in 2-3 hours, or take smaller doses several times a day.

What It Does: Helps with common cold, healing after surgery, produces collagen, heals burns, bleeding gums, red blood cell formation, shock and infection resistance and protects against cancer causing agents.

Health Benefits: Helps alcoholism, asthma, arteriosclerosis, arthritis, high cholesterol, colds, cystitis, hypoglycemia, heart disease, hepatitis, insect bites, scurvy, sinusitis, stress and tooth decay.

Sources: Citrus fruits, kiwis, berries, green and leafy vegetables, tomatoes, potatoes and sweet potatoes and rosehips.

Friends: All vitamins and minerals, especially calcium, magnesium and bioflavinoids.

Enemies: Cooking, water, light, oxygen and smoking.

Cautions: Nontoxic, but excessive doses may cause diarrhea, excess urination, skin rashes. Cut back doses if these symptoms occur.

Bioflavonoids

Rutin, Hesperidin (Water Soluble)
RDA N/A
Known as vitamin P, these are needed to absorb vitamin C. No RDA established, but most authorities say for each 500 mg of vitamin C, 100 mg of bioflavonoids should be taken.

What It Does: Prevents vitamin C from being destroyed by oxidation. Helps prevent bruising and builds resistance to infection.

Health Benefits: Helps asthma, bleeding gums, colds, eczema, edema, dizziness, hemorrhoids, high blood pressure, hypertension, miscarriages, rheumatic fever, rheumatism, ulcers, hot flushes due to menopause, if taken with vitamin C, and easy bruising.

Sources: Citrus fruits' white skin and segment membranes, buckwheat, blackberries, apricots, cherries and rosehips.

Friends: Vitamin C

Enemies: Unknown

Cautions: Nontoxic

Vitamin D

(Calciferol) (Fat Soluble) RDA 400
IU for adults
Known as "the sunshine vitamin" because ultraviolet rays act with skin oils to produce it. When taken internally it is absorbed with fats through the intestinal walls.
Vitamin D production stops after suntan. Many foods, especially dairy products, contain vitamin D supplements.

What It Does: Helps absorb vitamin A, calcium and phosphorus, strengthens bones and teeth, helps metabolism and slows premature aging.

Sources: Sunshine, sprouted seeds, mushrooms, sunflower seeds, egg yolks, milk, butter, fish oils and fish.

Friends: Vitamins A and C, choline, calcium and phosphorus.

Enemies: Air pollution and mineral oil.

Cautions: Do not use more than 25,000 IU daily for a long time. Signs of toxicity may be unusual thirst, sore eyes, skin irritation, diarrhea, vomiting and urinary urgency.

Vitamin E

(Tocopherol) (Fat Soluble) RDA
200 - 1,200
Unlike other fat soluble vitamins, vitamin E is only stored in the body for a short time, so daily supplementation is important. If using inorganic iron (ferrous sulfate) do not take with vitamin E, as it destroys vitamin E. Organic iron (ferious gluconate, peptonate, citrate or fumerate) complexes do not harm vitamin E. Pregnant, lactating women or those taking the birth control pill need more E, as do persons drinking chlorinated water. Strongly recommended for helping control hot flushes.

What It Does: A powerful antioxidant and anit-coagulant. Enhances effectiveness of vitamin A, alleviates fatigue, dilates blood vessels, improves circulation and strengthens capillary walls.

Health Benefits: Helps allergies, arteriosclerosis, baldness, blood clots, high cholesterol, diabetes, menopausal and menstrual problems, migraines, sinusitis, stress, sterility and varicose veins. Externally applied for burns, scars and wounds to increase healing.

Sources: Wheat germ, leafy green vegetables, whole grains, vegetable oils, soy beans and eggs.

Friends: Vitamins A, B-complex and C, manganese and selenium.

Enemies: Heat and cold, oxygen, iron, chlorine and mineral oil.

Cautions: Nontoxic

Vitamin F

(Unsaturated Fatty Acids) (Linoleic and Arachidonic) (Fat Soluble)
No RDA established but nutritional authorities suggest at least 1% of total calories should include these factors.

What It Does: Blood pressure normalizer, alleviates high cholesterol, combats heart disease, helps glandular activity, promotes healthy skin, hair and vital organs.

Health Benefits: Helps acne, allergies, baldness, asthma, high cholesterol, eczema, gallbladder and kidney problems, heart disease, leg ulcers, psoriasis, rheumatoid arthritis and weight problems.

Sources: Vegetable oils, wheat germ, flax seeds and oil, almonds, avocados, peanuts, soy beans and most nuts except cashews and Brazil nuts.

Friends: Vitamin E at mealtime.

Enemies: Heat, oxygen and saturated fats.

Cautions: Nontoxic, but excess can cause overweight.

Vitamin K

(Menadione) (Fat Soluble) K1 - K3
Measured in micrograms. No dietary allowance known, but adult intake of 300 mcg is recommended. Needed to form prothrombin, a blood-clotting chemical. Can be made by bacteria in the intestines.

What It Does: Helps prevent internal bleeding and hemorrhages and is important for liver function.

Health Benefits: Helps bruising, Celiac disease, colitis, gall stones, ulcers and preparation for childbirth.

Sources: Alfalfa, egg yolk, soy bean oil, kelp, leafy green vegetables, fish liver oils and safflower oil.

Friends: Unknown

Enemies: X-rays and radiation, aspirin, air pollution and mineral oil.

Cautions: Do not take more than 500 mcg of synthetic vitamin K.

Guide to Minerals

Calcium

RDA 800 - 1200 mg

Calcium and iron are the two minerals most deficient in the North American woman's diet. Calcium, magnesium and phosphorus work together. Most of the body's calcium is found in the teeth and bones. There must be two parts calcium to one part phosphorus. (Remember that animal products are high in phosphorus, so if you eat a lot, the balance may be upset.) Calcium and magnesium need to work together to promote cardiovascular health. Many supplements contain both in proper ratios. Dolomite, a natural source of calcium and magnesium, does not need vitamin D to assimilate. Look for a calcium supplement with vitamin D for added absorption.

What It Does: Aids tooth and bone formation, soothes the nerves, facilitates nerve transmission and helps to metabolize iron.

Health Benefits: Helps arthritis, backache, bone pain, foot and leg cramps, insomnia, hypoglycemia, menstrual cramps, PMS and menopause, nervousness, rheumatism and teenage growing pains.

Sources: Peanuts, walnuts, sunflower and sesame seeds, dried beans, green vegetables and milk products.

Friends: Vitamins A, C and D, iron, magnesium, manganese and phosphorus.

Enemies: Oxalic acid (rhubarb and chocolate), excess fat, phytic acid (grains) can all prevent absorption and use of calcium.

Cautions: Taking more than 2000 mg daily might lead to hypercalcemia. Many people use dairy products to increase their calcium, on top of an already high-protein, meat-based diet. Recent studies have shown that when people eat large amounts of protein, the body uses a great deal of calcium in the process of excreting the excess animal protein, a problem which does not occur with plant protein. If you are worried about calcium, just eat less animal products and more fresh green vegetables, grains, legumes and nuts and seeds.

Chlorine

RDA 500 mg

Chlorinated drinking water destroys vitamin E, and is not a good substitute for dietary sources or supplements.

What It Does: Regulates the blood's alkaline-acid balance, helps clean out wastes by aiding the liver and helps in production of hydrochloric acid for digestion. If you use table salt, you are probably getting enough.

Health Benefits: Helps digestion, stomach acidity and stiff joints.

Sources: Kelp, water cress, avocado, chard, cabbage, kale, celery, asparagus, cucumber, olives, tomatoes, turnip and saltwater fish.

Friends: Sodium and potassium.

Enemies: Unknown

Cautions: Do not take over 15 grams.

Chromium
RDA N/A
Most adults need about 90 mcg, but need increases with age.

What It Does: Works with insulin to metabolize sugar. Helps prevent high blood pressure and diabetes.

Sources: Nutritional yeast, cane sugar, corn oil, meat and shellfish.

Friends: Unknown

Enemies: Unknown

Cautions: Nontoxic

Cobalt
RDA N/A
A mineral that is part of vitamin B12 and must be obtained from diet.

What It Does: Aids in hemoglobin formation.

Sources: All green leafy vegetables and most animal and fish products.

Health Benefits: Anemia

Friends: Vitamin B12

Enemies: Sunlight, water, acids and alkalies, alcohol, estrogen and sleeping pills.

Cautions: Nontoxic. Vegetarians should look for cobalt in a supplement which also contains B12.

Copper
RDA 2 mg
Needed by the body to convert iron to hemoglobin. Most people rarely need to supplement.

What It Does: Aids in development of bones, brain, nerves, connective tissue, skin and hair color and healing processes.

Sources: Almonds, beans, peas, prunes, raisins, whole grains, green leafy vegetables, seafood and liver.

Friends: Iron and zinc.

Enemies: Unknown

Cautions: Toxicity rare, unless suffering from Wilson's disease.

Fluorine
RDA N/A
Added to many water supplies to reduce tooth decay.

What It Does: Strengthens teeth.

Health Benefits: Prevents tooth decay.

Sources: Carrots, garlic, sunflower seeds, fluoridated drinking water, seafood and gelatin.

Friends: Unknown

Enemies: Unknown

Cautions: 20 to 80 mg may be toxic.

Germanium
RDA N/A
A relatively new mineral.

What It Does: Helps build immune cells, gives energy and has rejuvenative properties.

Health Benefits: Helps anemia.

Sources: Garlic, aloe, comfrey, chlorella, ginseng and water cress.

Friends: Unknown
Enemies: Unknown
Cautions: Unknown

Iodine
RDA 150 mcg
Known for thyroid gland function.

What It Does: Helps with weight control by burning excess fat, boosts energy, helps mental function and promotes healthy skin, nails, teeth and hair.

Health Benefits: Helps cold hands and feet, dry hair, irritability, nervousness and obesity.

Sources: Kelp, dulse and sea vegetables, citrus fruits, artichokes, garlic, green leafy vegetables, pineapples, pears, seafood and egg yolks.

Friends: Unknown

Enemies: Nutrient-poor soil (Midwest) and food processing.

Cautions: Nontoxic if from natural sources. Iodine as a drug can be harmful if used incorrectly.

Iron
RDA 10 mg for males and 18 mg for females
Essential for the production of red blood cells. Only about 8% of total iron intake is absorbed. In one month, menstruating women lose about two times the iron that men do. The 4 gram supply in healthy bodies is recycled, mostly as hemoglobin, and replaced about every two months.

What It Does: Helps promote growth, resistance to disease, healthy skin tone. Helps prevent fatigue and iron-deficiency anemia.

Health Benefits: Helps alcoholism, anemia, colitis and menstrual problems.

Sources: Apricots, peaches, bananas, unrefined molasses, prunes, raisins, whole rye, nutritional yeast, sea vegetables, dry beans and lentils, liver and most meats.

Friends: Vitamins B12 and C, folic acid, copper and cobalt.

Enemies: Large quantities of coffee and tea may prevent absorption.

Cautions: Nontoxic for most adults, but excessive iron may be harmful for children. Many supplements contain ferrous sulfate, an inorganic form of iron which destroys vitamin E, so should not be taken within eight hours of each other.

Lithium
RDA N/A

What It Does: Helps transport sodium metabolism to brain, nerves and muscles.

Health Benefits: Reputed to be helpful for paranoid schizophrenia.

Sources: All sea vegetables and seafood.

Friends: Unknown
Enemies: Unknown
Cautions: Unknown

Magnesium
RDA 350 mg
Needed for better vitamin C, calcium, sodium, potassium and phosphorus metabolism. Magnesium is known as an anti-stress mineral. Needed when under stress, pregnant or lactating.

What It Does: Helps control depression and indigestion. Helps prevent heart disease, gall stones and calcium deposits in kidneys.

Health Benefits: Helps alcoholism, high cholesterol, depression, heart disease, kidney stones, prostate problems, stomach acidity, nervousness, sensitivity to noise, tooth decay and obesity.

Sources: Figs, lemons, grapefruit, yellow corn, almonds, nuts, seeds, green leafy vegetables, apples and whole grains.

Friends: Vitamins B6, C and D, calcium and phosphorus.

Enemies: Alcohol and diuretics.

Cautions: Do not take large amounts of magnesium, calcium and phosphorus over long periods, or toxicity can result.

Manganese

RDA N/A but some recommend 2.5 - 7 mg
Needed for digestion, reproduction and nervous system function.

What It Does: May improve memory, help with fatigue, irritability and improve muscle reflexes.

Health Benefits: Helps allergies, asthma, diabetes, fatigue and poor memory.

Sources: Nuts, green leafy vegetables, peas, beets, whole grains, blueberries, citrus fruits and egg yolks.

Friends: B-complex, E and calcium.

Enemies: Excess calcium and phosphorus may prevent absorption.

Cautions: Nontoxic, except for industrial sources.

Molybdenum

RDA N/A but some recommend 45 - 500 mcg
Needed for iron absorption, and carbohydrate and fat metabolism.

What It Does: Helps absorb iron.

Health Benefits: Helps anemia, copper poisoning and poor carbohydrate metabolism.

Sources: Leafy green vegetables, whole grains and legumes.

Friends: Unknown

Enemies: Unknown

Cautions: Toxicity rare. Most people do not need to supplement, as foods provide adequate amounts.

Phosphorus

RDA 800 - 1200 mg
Present in every cell, and essential to most body functions.

What It Does: Helps growth and repairs the body. Helps metabolize fats and starches, so provides fuel for energy. Promotes healthy teeth and gums. May help arthritis pain.

Health Benefits: Helps arthritis, stunted growth, stress and tooth and gum disease.

Sources: Whole grains, nuts, seeds and animal products.

Friends: Vitamins A and D, calcium, iron, manganese and magnesium.

Enemies: Excessive aluminum, magnesium and iron can inhibit the effectiveness of phosphorus.

Cautions: Excess phosphorus will upset mineral balance and cause calcium deficiency. Reduce intake of meat and other animal products as they are high in phosphorus. Avoid foods processed with phosphates in your diet.

Potassium
RDA 2000 - 2500 mg
Stress can cause a potassium deficiency, as can large amounts of coffee and alcohol.

What It Does: Sends oxygen to the brain, so helps thinking processes. Helps reduce blood pressure and dispose of body wastes.

Health Benefits: Helps acne, alcoholism, allergies, burns, colic in babies, diabetes, high blood pressure and heart disease.

Sources: Citrus fruits, green leafy vegetables, sunflower seeds, bananas, potatoes, whole grains and tomatoes.

Friends: Vitamin B6

Enemies: Alcohol, coffee, sugar and diuretics.

Cautions: More than 25 grams of potassium chloride may be toxic.

Selenium
RDA N/A, recommended 50 - 100 mcg
A powerful antioxidant together with vitamin E. Men have greater need for selenium in the reproductive system.

What It Does: Helps prevent aging and hardening of tissues by oxidation, may neutralize some carcinogens and prevent some cancers.

Health Benefits: Helps liver problems, impotence and mercury poisoning.

Sources: Nutritional yeast, wheat germ, bran, onions, garlic, mushrooms, tomatoes, broccoli, seafood, milk and eggs.

Friends: Vitamin E

Enemies: Food processing

Cautions: More than 200 mcg daily may be toxic.

Silicon
RDA N/A

What It Does: Helps build strong bones and immunity. Good for overall healing and strengthens hair, nails and teeth.

Health Benefits: Helps hair loss, irritation of mucous membranes, skin disorders and insomnia.

Sources: Flax seeds, oats, almonds, peanuts, sunflower seeds, apples, strawberries, grapes, sea vegetables, beets, onions and parsnips.

Friends: Unknown

Enemies: Unknown

Cautions: Unknown

Sodium
RDA 200 - 600 mg
Sodium and potassium are needed for normal growth. Too much sodium will deplete potassium and may cause high blood pressure.

What It Does: Helps prevent sunstroke, keeps nerves and muscles functioning.

Sources: Salt, carrots, beets, celery, artichokes, meats and seafood.

Friends: Unknown

Enemies: Unknown

Cautions: Over 14 grams of table

salt daily may be toxic. Avoid prepared foods as they contain too much sodium.

Sulfur
RDA N/A
Most protein foods have plenty of sulfur, so it is not necessary to supplement.

What It Does: Keeps oxygen balance for brain function, promotes healthy skin, hair and nails, and is part of tissue-building amino acids. Helps promote bile secretion in the liver and fight bacterial infections.

Health Benefits: Helps prevent heart attacks and high blood pressure.

Sources: Cruciferous vegetables, cabbage, broccoli, kale, turnips, radish, onions, celery, soy beans, water cress, eggs, fish and beef.

Friends: B-complex

Enemies: Unknown

Cautions: Nontoxic from organic sources, but large amounts of inorganic sulfur may be toxic.

Vanadium
RDA N/A

What It Does: May prevent formation of cholesterol in blood vessels.

Sources: Fish

Health Benefits: Helps prevents heart attacks.

Friends: Unknown

Enemies: Unknown

Cautions: Synthetic form may be toxic.

Zinc
RDA 15 mg

What It Does: Important for protein synthesis, regulating many body processes, enzyme systems and especially important for normalizing prostate gland in men. Excess sweating can cause a loss of zinc. Supplementation is recommended for most people, as processing and poor soils may result in low levels in normal food.

Health Benefits: Helps regain loss of taste, alcoholism, arteriosclerosis, baldness, cirrhosis, diabetes, healing wounds and injuries, lowering high cholesterol, infertility, impotence, menstrual and prostate problems, senility in the elderly and getting rid of white spots on fingernails.

Sources: Sprouted seeds, wheat bran and germ, pumpkin seeds, sunflower seeds, nutritional yeast, onions, nuts, green leafy vegetables, red meat, eggs and seafood.

Friends: Vitamin A, calcium and phosphorus.

Enemies: Unknown

Cautions: Nontoxic, unless food from galvanized containers is used in large amounts. Take more zinc of you are taking high B6. Alcoholics and diabetics also need more.

Part 2

Herbs and Herbal Combinations

*I*n North America, the use of herbs to promote health is now coming back into popularity. For almost 50 years, the ancient practice of healing and keeping healthy through herbs was considered backward and ineffective in light of the new science of pharmacology. However, for thousands of years people used botanical preparations to heal themselves. Many of the indigenous people around the world still know and use this wisdom, passed down through the generations. It is surprising that North American health practices are only now rediscovering the herbal traditions in healing.

You may be surprised to learn that about half the "wonder drugs" at the pharmacy are either derived from herbs, or are chemical imitations of substances found in plants. Common wild foxglove produces digitalis, a powerful heart medication, and the bark of the willow tree prompted the idea for the common aspirin. The ancients knew to put moldy bread on wounds to prevent infection, an early use of penicillin.

When using herbs as remedies for an ailment, remember that though herbs usually take a longer time to work than powerful pharmaceutical drugs, they have far fewer negative effects. Herbs often act on the source of the problem, not just the symptom, to promote health. However, it is still best to consult with an experienced herbologist if possible, especially for children, pregnant women or people with serious illnesses. About 1% of plants are poisonous, so it is best to buy preparations from trusted sources. A reliable source for herbal products is Nature Made. (See Resources section for more information.)

Courses on herbs are available now in many communities, and guided herbal nature walks are wonderful ways to learn about gathering and preparing your own medicinal preparations. But, for most busy North Americans, buying ready-made preparations is a safer and more realistic route.

Guide to Herbs

Alfalfa

Common plant used for cattle fodder, but long known for its rich mineral and nutrient content.

Parts Used: Leaves, flowers, petals and sprouts.

Medicinal Properties: Aids in assimilating protein, fats and carbohydrates, boosts appetite, aids water retention and relieves constipation. Good for pregnant and nursing women. Helps detoxify the liver. Relieves painful arthritis and rheumatism.

How to Use: Capsules, tablets or dry powder mixed with food or liquid. A tea or fresh sprouts in salads or sandwiches.

Cautions: People with lupus or auto-immune disorders should avoid alfalfa.

Aloe Vera

Succulent desert plant often used as house plant, known for quick healing of burns.

Parts Used: Leaves or the gel

Medicinal Properties: An excellent healer of sunburns, minor burns, bug bites and mild skin irritations. Internally, aloe vera works as a laxative and promotes healing. A good remedy for hemorrhoids and colon cleansing. Promotes immunity.

How to Use: Internally, capsules, juice or gel, as directed. Externally, the gel may be used liberally.

Cautions: Pregnant women, children and the elderly should not take aloe vera internally.

Angelica

Versatile. Good for indigestion and stomach upsets.

Parts Used: Herb, root and seeds.

Medicinal Properties: Resists toxins. Helps with gas, colic and heartburn. Promotes secretion of phlegm from respiratory system. Tea taken hot is reputed to quickly break up a cold. Reduces discomfort caused by rheumatism and relieves menstrual cramps. A remedy for skin lice.

How to Use: Internally, extract, as directed. Externally, rub liquid on affected areas.

Cautions: Do not use during pregnancy. Large doses can affect blood pressure, heart and respiration.

Anise

Since the Middle Ages, sweet licorice anise tea has increased milk in nursing mothers.

Parts Used: Seeds

Medicinal Properties: Promotes digestion and relieves nausea and gas. Good for colds and coughs. Stimulates breast milk production.

How to Use: Crush seeds into powder, pour boiling water over and steep to make tea.

Cautions: None known.

Arnica

Healers have used this herb for pain relief, but modern herbalists feel it is too strong to be taken internally, so creams and ointments are made.

Parts Used: Flower and root.

Medicinal Properties: Relieves muscle pain, joint inflammation and athletic injuries. Heals skin irritations and wounds.

How to Use: There are many good salves or ointments on the market.

Cautions: Do not apply arnica on broken skin, or take internally unless under supervision of a licensed practitioner.

Astragalus

An ancient Chinese herb creating excitement now because of its immune enhancing properties.

Parts Used: Root

Medicinal Properties: Promotes resistance to disease. May improve blood pressure and digestion.

How to Use: Internally, by capsule, as directed.

Cautions: For serious illness, especially chemotherapy, do not use without supervision of licensed practitioner.

Bayberry Bark

A versatile Native American plant.

Parts Used: Root bark

Medicinal Properties: An astringent and mild stimulant. Helps clear congestion due to colds. Soothes varicose veins and hemorrhoids.

How to Use: Internally, take capsules as directed. Extract, mix prescribed number of drops in water. Powder, mix with water. For sore throats, use mouthwash, as directed. Externally, rub liquid mixture on hemorrhoids or varicose veins.

Cautions: Large doses may cause vomiting.

Bilberry

Folk remedy for vision problems, especially night blindness.

Parts Used: Leaves and berries.

Medicinal Properties: Helps preserve eyesight and prevent eye damage. Similar in nature to insulin. Good for diarrhea and liver and stomach conditions.

How to Use: Internally, capsules or extract, mix drops in water, as directed.

Cautions: The leaves can be poisonous if used in excess.

Black Cohosh

Native American plant used by indigenous people for pain, inflammation and female problems.

Parts Used: Root

Medicinal Properties: Relieves swelling and soreness of neuralgia and rheumatism. Helpful for poisonous bites, sinusitis and asthma. Helps lower blood pressure, cholesterol and mucus levels. A relaxant, promotes labor and eases delivery.

How to Use: Internally, capsules or tincture, as directed.

Cautions: None known.

Black Walnut

Known for being high in manganese, which is good for brain and nerves.

Parts Used: Bark, leaves and fruit.

Medicinal Properties: Helps relieve constipation and diarrhea. Helps treat tuberculosis, heal mouth sores, soothe skin problems and fight bacterial and fungal infections. Expels internal parasites.

How to Use: Internally, take drops in water, as directed. Externally, rub ointment on skin, as directed.

Cautions: None known.

Blessed Thistle

Popular folk cure for menstrual cycle problems.

Parts Used: Flower, leaves, root and seeds

Medicinal Properties: Regulates appetite and menstrual cycle. Useful for liver problems, fevers and stopping bleeding. Also useful for increasing milk production in mothers.

How to Use: Capsules or drops, as directed.

Cautions: Avoid during pregnancy.

Blue Cohosh

A well-known relaxant for the female reproductive system.

Parts Used: Root

Medicinal Properties: Helps low blood pressure, cleanses blood and causes sweating. Can prevent or relieve muscle cramps, colic, diabetes, nervousness and rheumatism.

How to Use: Capsules, as directed.

Cautions: Avoid in early stages of pregnancy.

Blue Vervain

A herb best known for its purifying abilities.

Parts Used: Leaves, root and stems.

Medicinal Properties: Good for asthma, epilepsy, stress and upset nerves. Helps relieve gas, diarrhea, colds, fevers and flu, female problems, headaches and pneumonia. Regulates blood circulation and helps expel phlegm from lungs and throat.

How to Use: Capsules, as directed.

Cautions: Do not take if pregnant.

Boneset

Used by the North American indigenous peoples for severe flu, its uses were passed on to early settlers.

Parts Used: Leaves and tops.

Medicinal Properties: Reduces fevers, promotes sweating and aids constipation as it is a mild laxative. Used in treatment of rheumatism.

How to Use: Capsules, as directed.

Cautions: None known.

Borage

Ancient herb with newly discovered properties. An excellent source of gamma linoleic acid (GLA) used to treat PMS symptoms. A delightful herb to grow. The blue flowers have a sweet cucumber taste, good in salads with nasturtiums.

Parts Used: Seeds, leaves and tops.

Medicinal Properties: Good for increasing breast milk production, clearing phlegm from lungs, treating ulcers and soothing nerves.

How to Use: Internally, extract or capsules, as directed.

Cautions: None known.

Buchu

An aromatic South African plant used for healing by natives for over 400 years.

Parts Used: Leaves

Medicinal Properties: Good for bladder infections, cystitis and digestive disorders.

How to Use: Capsules or drops, as directed.

Cautions: Do not use for kidney problems, as medical attention is essential, and buchu can be irritating to kidneys.

Burdock

Called "Nature's blood purifier."

Parts Used: Leaves, stems, root and seeds.

Medicinal Properties: A blood purifier that helps boils, eczema and other skin problems. Good for gout, arthritic swelling and kidney irritation. Relieves snake bites.

How to Use: Internally, capsules or extract, as directed. Externally, apply to inflamed area.

Cautions: None known.

Butcher's Broom

Popular in Europe for swelling in the legs.

Parts Used: Seeds and tops.

Medicinal Properties: Good for varicose veins, hemorrhoids and restless leg syndrome. Its anti-inflammatory action is good for arthritic swelling. Improves circulation and reduces edema.

How to Use: Capsules or extract, as directed.

Cautions: None known.

Calendula

An attractive common yellow garden flower with wonderful healing properties.

Parts Used: Essential oil

Medicinal Properties: Soothes burns and helps wounds to heal. Helps reduce fever if taken internally. Relieves menstrual cramps. Can help some skin diseases caused by virus, such as shingles.

How to Use: Internally, tea from dried herb or extract, as directed. Externally, apply oil or salve directly on affected part.

Cautions: Do not use if pregnant.

Caraway

Another popular cooking herb with beneficial health effects.

Parts Used: Seeds

Medicinal Properties: Aids digestion and appetite, coughs and colds. Relieves colic in babies, gas and other stomach disorders. Aids production of breast milk.

How to Use: Extract, as directed, or chew or make tea from the seeds.

Cautions: Children should have tea or extract, not seeds.

Cascara Sagrada

Known for its laxative properties.

Parts Used: Dried bark.

Medicinal Properties: Relieves constipation. Good for hemorrhoids and gall stones, increases secretion of bile. Has a mild, yet effective action.

How to Use: Capsules, as directed.

Cautions: Overdosing can cause diarrhea and cramps.

Catnip

Useful for humans as a mild sedative, though it has the opposite effect on cats.

Parts Used: Whole herb

Medicinal Properties: Relieves stress, soothes the nerves and is a digestive aid for gas and diarrhea. Good for colic in young children. Controls fever by promoting perspiration. A good sleeping aid.

How to Use: Capsules, as directed.

Cautions: None known.

Cayenne Pepper Fruit

A popular hot spice that has medicinal uses.

Parts Used: Fruit (Capsicum is the most important constituent.)

Medicinal Properties: Good to take with other herbs as it improves circulation and aids digestion. Good for cold symptoms. Helps inflammation. Improves health of heart, lungs, kidneys, pancreas, spleen and stomach.

How to Use: Internally, capsules or tea, as directed. Externally, liniment applied on affected parts.

Cautions: Do not use with hemorrhoids or for gastro-intestinal problems. High doses can cause kidney damage and gastroenteritis. Do not use ointment on broken skin.

Chamomile

An old-fashioned calming remedy.

Parts Used: Flowers and herb.

Medicinal Properties: Relieves hysteria, nightmares and nervous problems. A digestive aid for weak stomachs which boosts appetite. Also good for rheumatism, back pain and certain skin irritations.

How to Use: Internally, capsules, extract or tea, as directed. Externally, apply extract to skin irritations.

Cautions: Do not use if allergic to ragweed, as chamomile is a member of the daisy family.

Chaparral

Known as "Nature's excellent antibiotic." Native Americans taught settlers about this herb. It contains an antioxidant which can help prevent some cancerous tumors and premature aging.

Parts Used: Leaves and stems.

Medicinal Properties: Helps fight infection, acne, arthritis, skin blemishes and warts. Good for liver, lymphatic and digestive disorders. Rids body of excess water, reduces inflammation and helps stop diarrhea. Protects from the sun.

How to Use: Internally, capsules and extract, as directed. Externally, apply extract on injured parts.

Cautions: None known.

Chickweed

A weed long used in folk medicine.

Parts Used: Whole herb

Medicinal Properties: Helps with weight control. Good for respiratory and digestive systems. Excellent remedy for tumors, hemorrhoids and swollen testes. Healing and soothing for bruises, irritations, eczema and other skin problems.

How to Use: Internally, capsules, as directed. Externally, ointment as needed.

Cautions: None known.

Cloves

Spice from China, used for over 2000 years, thought to be aphrodisiac.

Parts Used: Dried buds of clove tree.

Medicinal Properties: Good reputation for relieving toothaches and controlling vomiting. Clove oil is highly antiseptic, so good to take on camping trips.

How to Use: Oil, for toothache, rub on affected area. For vomiting, mix 2 drops of oil in cup of water and drink.

Cautions: None known.

Comfrey

Known as "knitbone" for its healing properties, this herb has come under some controversy lately because it contains some compounds that may cause liver disease if taken for a prolonged period of time.

Parts Used: Roots and leaves.

Medicinal Properties: Promotes healing of skin wounds and broken bones. Relieves skin irritations, ulcers, coughs and catarrh.

How to Use: Internally, not recommended except under the supervision of a licensed practitioner. Externally, as an ointment.

Cautions: To protect breastfeeding babies, do not use ointments which contain comfrey for sore nipples.

Cornsilk

Folk remedy for bladder problems.

Parts Used: The long silky fibers from a cob of corn.

Medicinal Properties: Helps inflammation in the bladder, kidney and urethra. Good for any conditions due to uric acid build-up. Helps bedwetting and enlarged prostate gland.

How to Use: Make a tea of the silk and drink.

Cautions: None known.

Cranberry

Organically grown berries have health benefits for the urinary tract.

Parts Used: Berries

Medicinal Properties: Natural cranberry juice and berries seem to prevent bacteria from adhering to the urinary tract. Also good for asthma and anxiety.

How to Use: Fresh organic juice, or capsules, as directed.

Cautions: The bottled juice in supermarkets is highly processed with heavy sugar content, and is not recommended.

Damiana

A folk remedy for impotence.

Parts Used: Leaves

Medicinal Properties: Reputed to increase libido. Helps relieve constipation, bedwetting and depression. Boosts energy and balances female hormones.

How to Use: Capsules or extract, as directed.

Cautions: Damiana can interfere with iron absorption.

Dandelion

A weed high in iron, calcium and other vitamins and minerals.

Parts Used: Root and leaves. Wine has been made with flowers.

Medicinal Properties: Strengthens kidneys and bladder, removes excess fluids and toxins, helps gall stones and jaundice and anemia.

How to Use: Capsules or extract, as directed.

Cautions: None known.

Devil's Claw

Used in Europe and Africa for over 250 years, it is just being "discovered" in North America as an effective anti-inflammatory and painkiller, especially for arthritis.

Parts Used: Roots and leaves.

Medicinal Properties: A good blood cleanser, anti-inflammatory and painkiller against arthritis, gout and rheumatism. Good for liver and kidney disorders.

How to Use: Capsules, as directed.

Cautions: Do not use if pregnant.

Dill

Aromatic herb, traditionally used by Scandinavians in cooking.

Parts Used: Leaves and seeds.

Medicinal Properties: Soothes indigestion and promotes appetite. Helps promote breast milk production.

How to Use: Make tea with fresh leaves and stems or seeds. Grind seeds and make tea, or chew seeds.

Cautions: None known.

Dong Quai

Popular Chinese herb, known as "women's ginseng." A plant rich in many vitamins including B12.

Parts Used: Root

Medicinal Properties: Most noted for help with female reproductive system, specifically for PMS, hot flushes in menopause and menstrual irregularity. Helps bring down high blood pressure.

How to Use: Capsules, as directed.

Cautions: Do not use if you have heavy menstrual flow or during pregnancy.

Echinacea

Very popular immune system booster, known for its ability to help the body resist disease. American Purple coneflower introduced to settlers by indigenous people. Try to find capsules that use organically grown herb.

Parts Used: Leaves, dried rhizome and root.

Medicinal Properties: Helps boost immune response. Works best in prevention and treatment of some viral, bacterial and fungal infections. Good defense, in advance, for colds and flu. Good for the lymphatic system and liver, boils, blood poisoning, and snake and spider bites.

How to Use: Extract or capsules, as directed.

Cautions: The medicinal properties of Echinacea are easily destroyed. If you taste a tingle when drinking the extract, it is still potent; if not, try a new supply.

Ephedra

Known as ma huang in Chinese medicine.

Parts Used: Roots and twigs, or stems.

Medicinal Properties: A stimulant and decongestant, good for asthma and upper respiratory infections, headaches, allergies and a stuffy nose.

How to Use: Capsules or tea, as directed.

Cautions: Do not use if pregnant, or if high blood pressure, heart disease, enlarged prostrate, diabetes or thyroid problems, except on advice of licensed practitioner.

Eucalyptus

Oil of eucalyptus is a familiar smell in cold and flu preparations.

Parts Used: Oil extracted from leaves.

Medicinal Properties: Good antiseptic and expectorant, so helps with cold, flu and stiffness or swelling of arthritis.

How to Use: Externally only, do not apply to broken skin.

Cautions: None known.

Evening Primrose

Very popular lately, but used for centuries by indigenous American people.

Parts Used: Bark, leaves and seeds.
Medicinal Properties:
Known for being excellent source of essential fatty acids (EFAs). Good for female problems such as cramps, PMS, hot flushes and heavy bleeding. Also good for anxiety, reducing high blood pressure and maintaining healthy skin.

How to Use: Capsules, as directed. Look for capsules naturally preserved with vitamin E.

Cautions: None known.

Eyebright

As its name suggests, this popular herb has helped people with eye problems for centuries. Look for capsules with no additives, preferably organically grown in Europe.

Parts Used: Leaves

Medicinal Properties: Helps protect and maintain eye health. May relieve itchy eyes.

How to Use: Internally, capsules or tea, as directed. Externally, an eyewash, as directed.

Cautions: None known.

Fennel

A licorice-flavored herb with soothing properties. This plant grows as a tall weed in North America.

Parts Used: Whole herb

Medicinal Properties: Helps normalize appetite and control weight. Good for gout, gas and acid stomach. Helps conditions of the kidneys, liver and spleen.

How to Use: Internally, extract, as directed or seeds can be crushed and made into tea. Externally, apply oil to affected parts to relieve rheumatic and arthritic pain.

Cautions: Unknown

Fenugreek

Dating back to ancient Egyptian days, this plant has enjoyed popularity over the centuries, and is still recognized as an effective remedy for a variety of ailments.

Parts Used: Seeds

Medicinal Properties: Good for all mucous conditions, coughs, bronchitis, fevers, sore throats and inflammation of stomach and intestines. Also works as a bulk laxative and helps lower blood sugar.

How to Use: Internally, capsules or tablets, as directed or as gargle for sore throat. Externally, ground seeds can be applied as poultice, mixed with warm water, to painful parts.

Cautions: Unknown

Feverfew

Although modern herbalists are rediscovering this herb as a good treatment for migraine headaches, it has a long history as an effective folk remedy for a number of conditions.

Parts Used: Whole herb

Medicinal Properties: May prevent and ease migraine headaches. Relieves dizziness and menstrual cramps.

How to Use: Capsules, as directed.

Cautions: None known.

Fo-Ti

Famous Chinese rejuvenating tonic.

Parts Used: Root

Medicinal Properties: Helps memory, stimulates endocrine glands which strengthens the body, lowers cholesterol and may help prevent cancer.

How to Use: Internally, capsules, as directed.

Cautions: None known.

Garlic

Common kitchen herb, used by ancient Egyptians for its antibiotic properties, and also known as "Russian penicillin."

Parts Used: Bulb

Medicinal Properties: Natural antibiotic, bacteriostatic and antiviral. Stimulates digestion, good for asthma and whooping cough, can reduce high blood pressure and high cholesterol and even destroy some types of cancer cells.

How to Use: Internally, odorless capsules (avoids strong breath) as directed or, raw or cooked cloves in cooking. Externally, oil for aches, earaches or sprains.

Cautions: Do not eat more than 10 raw cloves a day, or you could have a toxic or allergic reaction. Do not use if breastfeeding, as it can cause colic in babies.

Gentian

A bitter herb used in tea to rejuvenate people suffering from exhaustion, stress and chronic fatigue.

Parts Used: Root

Medicinal Properties: Acts powerfully against exhaustion and debilitation from chronic illness. Increases a poor appetite and poor digestion.

How to Use: Tea made from the roots, as directed.

Cautions: Good for a "jump start", but should only be used in small quantities for a short time.

Ginger

Another common kitchen herb with many useful properties.

Parts Used: Root, fresh or dried and powdered.

Medicinal Properties: Good remedy for nausea, upset stomach, indigestion, cramps and diarrhea. Good for morning sickness, motion sickness and bronchitis and coughs. An anti-inflammatory, promotes healing of minor burns and skin inflammations and helps absorb toxins.

How to Use: Internally, capsules or extract, as directed. Externally, use drops mixed with vegetable oil and apply to inflamed parts.

Cautions: None known.

Ginkgo

Known as Ginkgo biloba, this herb has had a rise in popularity for its effects on the brain, memory and eyesight.

Parts Used: Leaves

Medicinal Properties: Good for memory, concentration, hearing and vision. Helps senility, dizziness, hemorrhoids, tinnitus and heart and kidney disorders. May help prevent cancer, slow aging process and help symptoms of Alzheimer's disease. Increases circulation and blood flow in the capillaries.

How to Use: Internally, standardized capsules or tablets, as directed.

Cautions: No known side effects have been found, so long-term use seems safe.

Ginseng (Panax)

Ancient Chinese herb popular in the Far East and Europe for hundreds of years. Panax is considered true ginseng, grown in Korea and North America, though the North American type is not as strong.

Parts Used: Root

Medicinal Properties: Seems effective in increasing mental and physical endurance. Helps body cope with stress, reduces cholesterol, helps protect from cancer, is useful for menopause symptoms, increases energy and generally normalizes body functions.

How to Use: Internally, capsules or powder, as directed.

Cautions: Ginseng Panax may be too stimulating for some people, so early in the day is best time to use. Do not take at the same time as vitamin C, as it interferes with ginseng's absorption. People with high blood pressure should check with licensed practitioner before using.

Ginseng (Siberian)

This is not true ginseng, though related, and it has many of the same properties. Often used by Russian athletes.

Parts Used: Roots

Medicinal Properties: Helps with menstrual and menopause problems, stress, infections, high cholesterol, high blood pressure and insomnia.

How to Use: Internally, capsules, extract or liquid, as directed.

Cautions: None known.

Goldenseal

An old and wide-spread herb with powerful healing qualities that is enjoying great popularity as modern health practitioners find many therapeutic uses for it.

Parts Used: Root

Medicinal Properties: A natural antibiotic good for most infections, especially when taken with echinacea. Helps digestion and constipation. Mouthwash of goldenseal can prevent gum disease. Can be used in a douche for vaginal infections. Used with myrrh, it is good for ulcers, or with gotu kola, good for the brain. Aids inflammation of the mucous membranes.

How to Use: Internally, capsules, extract or powder as directed. Externally, douche, as directed.

Cautions: People with high blood pressure should not use. Do not use during pregnancy. Do not use for more than two weeks. Eating fresh plant can cause mucous tissue inflammation.

Gotu Kola

Used in India and China, this herb is good for improving circulation, stress and fatigue related ailments.

Parts Used: Nuts, root and seeds.

Medicinal Properties: Aids circulatory system. Rejuvenating, it strengthens the heart and liver. Good for mental problems and aids memory. Helps high blood pressure, sore throats, tonsillitis, fevers, strengthening veins and capillaries, hepatitis, measles and rheumatism. Can treat phlebitis and leg cramps. Very good for people confined to bed. Aids recovery after childbirth.

How to Use: Capsules and extract, as directed.

Cautions: Do not use during pregnancy, or if thyroid is overactive.

Guar Gum

A popular additive to healthy low-fat dressings, as it makes a good thickener.

Parts Used: Leaves and seeds.

Medicinal Properties: Helps reduce cholesterol and aid constipation.

How to Use: In cooking, to thicken or mix with water, as directed.

Cautions: None known.

Hawthorn

The berries are rich in bioflavonoids, and were used in Europe as a tonic for the heart.

Parts Used: Berries and leaves.

Medicinal Properties: Helps burn off excess calories. Improves circulation and cardiovascular health.

How to Use: Capsules, as directed.

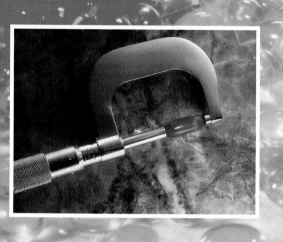

Modern production and testing methods ensure the highest standards

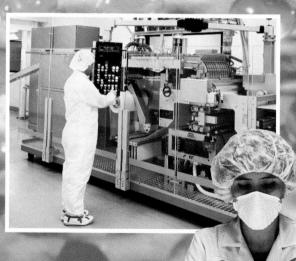

hotos courtesy Pharmative
lission Hills, CA

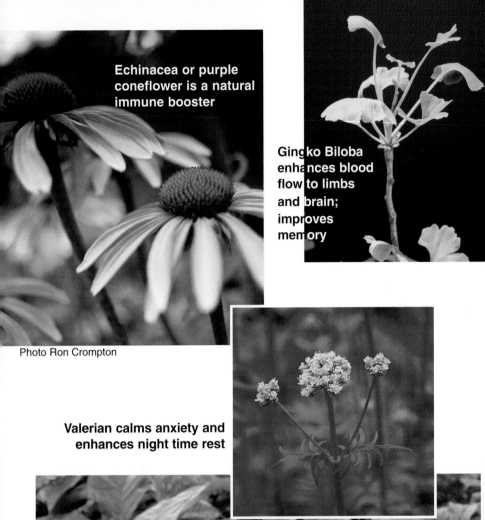

Echinacea or purple coneflower is a natural immune booster

Gingko Biloba enhances blood flow to limbs and brain; improves memory

Photo Ron Crompton

Valerian calms anxiety and enhances night time rest

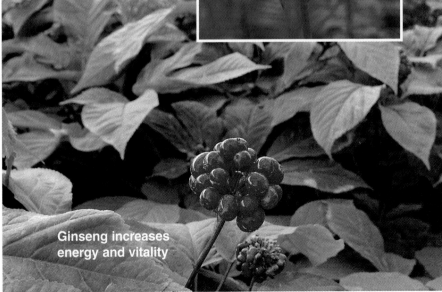

Ginseng increases energy and vitality

Photo courtesy of Atkins Ginseng Farms, Waterford ON

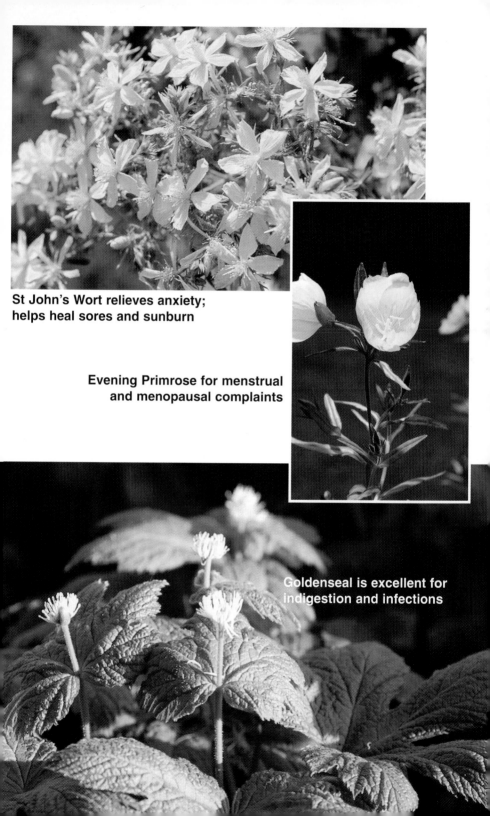

St John's Wort relieves anxiety;
helps heal sores and sunburn

Evening Primrose for menstrual
and menopausal complaints

Goldenseal is excellent for
indigestion and infections

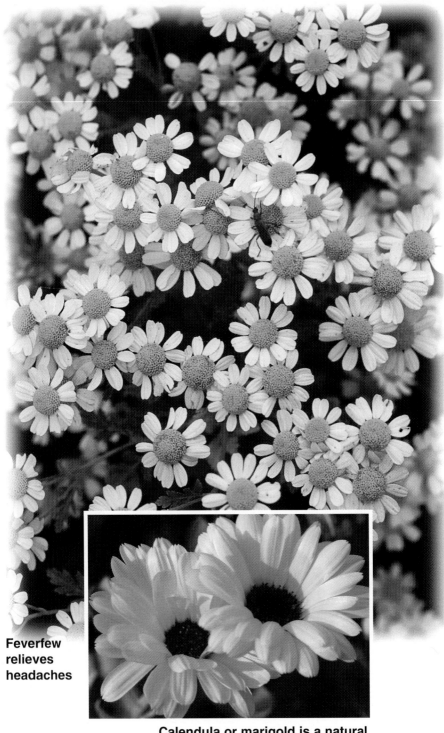

Feverfew relieves headaches

Calendula or marigold is a natural healer of skin conditions

Cautions: Some highly concentrated forms should be used on advice of licensed practitioner, though most products are quite safe.

Hops

Known most commonly for its use in beer making, hops' rich B vitamin content gives it many more practical and beneficial uses.

Parts Used: Flower cones

Medicinal Properties: Powerful yet safe sedative. Decreases craving for alcohol and improves appetite. Good for heart, stomach and liver, nervousness, pain, toothaches, earaches and stress.

How to Use: Young sprouts of wild hops make a pleasant tea.

Cautions: None known.

Horehound

A bitter, strong herb which was once made into Horehound Candy used for coughs.

Parts Used: Whole herb

Medicinal Properties: Relieves congestion, coughs, colds and gas. Promotes sweating and aids water retention.

How to Use: Internally, extract, as directed.

Cautions: None known.

Horse Chestnut

In folk medicine, carrying a fruit of this tree in your pocket can cure arthritis.

Parts Used: Bark and seeds.

Medicinal Properties: Reduces fever and cold symptoms, swelling

of varicose veins and hemorrhoids. Traditionally used as sunscreen. Promotes sweating.

How to Use: Externally, commercial preparations, as directed.

Cautions: Coating on seeds can be toxic, so peel them.

Horseradish

Do not be fooled by this member of the mustard family's small white flowers. Though it is attractive, its taste is quite bitter.

Parts Used: Root

Medicinal Properties: Soothing to respiratory system and may help rheumatism.

How to Use: Internally, grated root mixed with honey and warm water for coughs. Tablets, as directed. Externally, make poultice with cornstarch and apply.

Cautions: May cause diarrhea and heavy sweating if used in large quantities.

Horsetail

Long used in China and Europe, this common weed looks like miniature fir trees.

Parts Used: Leaves and stems.

Medicinal Properties: Rich in silica, it increases calcium absorption. Improves skin condition and strengthens bone, hair, nails and teeth. A diuretic that helps with kidney stones.

How to Use: Internally, capsules or tablets, as directed. Externally, used in beauty preparations.

Cautions: None known.

Huckleberry

A common forest plant with beneficial qualities. Edible berries are found either dark blue, semi-flat and shiny, or red in West Coast forests.

Parts Used: Whole plant

Medicinal Properties: Lowers blood sugar levels and relieves inflammation. Good for diabetes, kidney, bladder, sinusitis and ulcers.

How to Use: Internally, tablets or capsules, as directed.

Cautions: None known.

Hyssop

A good herb for treating the common cold.

Parts Used: Leaves and stems.

Medicinal Properties: A remedy for coughs, colds and sore throats. Improves appetite and relieves gas.

How to Use: Internally, dried herb or capsules, as directed.

Cautions: Consult licensed practitioner if using for more than two weeks.

Irish Moss

This herb is actually a seaweed with rich nutrient content.

Parts Used: Whole plant

Medicinal Properties: Effective in treatment of thyroid and colon disorders, and obesity.

How to Use: Internally, powder, in food or tablets or capsules, as directed. Externally, cosmetic products, as directed.

Cautions: None known.

Jasmine

A popluar addition to herbal teas, hailing from the Orient.

Parts Used: Flowers

Medicinal Properties: Calming and a possible aphrodisiac.

How to Use: Brewed into tea, fragrant and pleasant.

Cautions: None known.

Juniper Berries

In the Middle Ages, these berries were burned in homes where there was plague, offering an antiseptic smoke to help prevent the spread of disease.

Parts Used: Ripe dry berries

Medicinal Properties: Digestive problems, gastro-intestinal infections, cramps, kidney and bladder diseases. Also good for general inflammations, gout and other arthritic conditions. Helps rid body of excess water.

How to Use: Internally, extract or tea, as directed.

Cautions: Do not use if pregnant.

Kava Kava

Polynesians used this plant root to make a popular beverge.

Parts Used: Root

Medicinal Properties: Good for insomnia and nervousness as it promotes sleep and relaxation. Helps rid body of excess water.

How to Use: Internally, extract, as directed.

Cautions: Long-term use may cause liver damage, so use sparingly.

Kelp

High in calcium, sulfur, iodine, silicon and vitamin K, it is usually ground into powder and added to vegetable salt products or pressed into tablets.

Parts Used: Leaves

Medicinal Properties: Excellent for reproductive organs, blood vessels walls and the thyroid gland. Good for goiters, nerves, nails and hair.

How to Use: Kelp powder in cooking, or tablets, as directed.

Cautions: None known.

Lady's Mantle

Believed to keep women young and beautiful.

Parts Used: Leaves and stems.

Medicinal Properties: Promotes healing and menstrual regularity, stops bleeding, reduces vaginal irritation and improves appetite.

How to Use: Internally, tea, as directed. Externally, extract, as douche, as directed.

Cautions: None known.

Lavender

Popular garden plant, known for its tranquil fragrance.

Parts Used: Leaves, stems and flowers.

Medicinal Properties: Relaxing, good for headaches, anxiety and stomach gas.

How to Use: Externally, drops of oil in bath, or on handkerchief for smelling.

Cautions: None known.

Lemon Balm

An easy-to-grow plant of the mint family with a pleasant lemon smell.

Parts Used: Leaves and stems.

Medicinal Properties: Anti-viral, antibacterial and antispasmodic. Tones the stomach, calms the nerves and aids digestion.

How to Use: Internally, brew as a pleasant tea. Externally, leaves applied help to heal wounds.

Cautions: None known.

Licorice

A hormone balancer and natural cortisone. Popular for candy, though most commercial products are artificial and do not have medicinal properties of the root.

Parts Used: Dried root

Medicinal Properties: Soothing benefits for the stomach and for urinary tract infections. Reduces pain from ulcers, helps break up congestion from colds, soothes sore throats, and relieves pain and stiffness of arthritis. Used for hypoglycemia, adrenal glands and stress. May help stop growth of cancerous tumors and prevent tooth decay.

How to Use: Capsules or tea, as directed.

Cautions: Avoid if you have high blood pressure. Since it causes water retention, women should not use during PMS.

Lobelia

Known as Indian tobacco.

Parts Used: Leaves, flowers, seeds and stems.

Medicinal Properties: Good for fevers, hepatitis, meningitis, pneumonia, whooping cough, pleurisy, and peritonitis. Both a relaxant and a stimulant. Helps alcoholism and smoking. Aids in hormone production and reduces heart palpitations.

How to Use: Internally, capsules, as directed.

Cautions: Consult licensed practitioner for supervision.

Lungwort

Named because its leaf resembles a lung, this herb has amazing healing benefits for the respiratory system.

Parts Used: Leaves and stems.

Medicinal Properties: Helps with chest congestion due to colds, irritated throats and diarrhea.

How to Use: Dried herb as tea, as directed.

Cautions: See licensed practitioner if cough lasts longer than two weeks.

Marshmallow

This herb has a long history of use in Europe, and its properties have now been recognized in North America.

Parts Used: Whole herb.

Medicinal Properties: Good for inflammation and irritation of digestive, urinary, and respiratory systems. Good for coughs and colds. Has an overall soothing effect on body.

How to Use: Capsules or dried herb, as directed.

Cautions: None known.

Milk Thistle

In Europe, this herb has been a popular liver tonic, and now North Americans are discovering its beneficial qualities.

Parts Used: Fruit, leaves and seeds.

Medicinal Properties: Rejuvenates liver and protects from poisons, helps produce bile and breaks down fats and helps heal psoriasis. Helps recovery from alcohol, drug or chemical pollution. Good for smokers, or those exposed to smoke or pollutants.

How to Use: Capsules, with optimal flavonoid level of 80%, as directed.

Cautions: None known.

Milkweed

Used for its ability to clean the lungs and stimulate perspiration.

Parts Used: Root

Medicinal Properties: Good for asthma, bronchitis, rheumatism and arthritis, bowel and stomach complaints, gall stones and female problems.

How to Use: Capsules, as directed.

Cautions: Caution administering to children and people over 55.

Mullein

It grows by the roadside with a tall spike, small yellow flowers and soft silver-grey leaves.

Parts Used: Leaves and flowers.

Medicinal Properties: A pain reliever and glandular rebuilder. Good for coughs and colds, hay fever, shortness of breath and hemorrhoids.

How to Use: Dried herb or extract, as directed.

Cautions: None known.

Mustard

A large family of herbs, often grown in the Orient for greens, cooked or raw.

Parts Used: Ground up seeds of black and white variety.

Medicinal Properties: Increases blood flow to arthritic areas. Relieves joint pain and sciatics.

How to Use: Classic mustard plaster, as directed.

Cautions: Do not use undiluted oil, as it can be irritating.

Myrrh

This herbs is a treasured folk remedy for everything from fleas to muscle pains.

Parts Used: Leaves

Medicinal Properties: Appetite stimulator and digestive aid. Mouthwash for general gum and oral health. Relief from stomach flu. Good for bronchial and lung diseases.

How to Use: Dried herb or extract, as directed.

Cautions: Do not use during pregnancy or if you have kidney disease. High doses over a long time can be dangerous. Best to check with licensed practitioner.

Nettle

Found in North America and Europe, it has many purposes. In Russia, women use the tea as a rinse for shiny hair.

Parts Used: Roots and leaves.

Medicinal Properties: Relieves asthma, hay fever and other allergies. Lowers blood sugar. Good for iron production of red blood cells, diarrhea, dysentery, hemorrhoids and urinary disorders. Helps normalize menstrual flow and cure vaginal infections.

How to Use: Internally, capsules, dried herb or extract, as directed. Fresh herb, harvest leaves and stems without skin contact, and boil in water and drink as tea, and/or eat as cooked green.

Cautions: Harvesting fresh herb may cause painful sting if herb makes contact with skin. Cooking for five minutes destroys sting.

Oat Fiber

This has been popular in North America in recent years as a way to reduce cholesterol.

Parts Used: Seeds, stems and leaves.

Medicinal Properties: Rich source of B vitamins. Helps gas and upset stomach, lowers cholesterol and aids skin conditions and hemorrhoids.

How to Use: Internally, eat oats for breakfast or extract, as directed. Externally, straw may be made into bath preparation for hemorrhoids.

Cautions: None known.

Oregon Grape

The early settlers in North America used these berries to make a tart grape jelly that was full of vitamins and minerals.

Parts Used: Fruit

Medicinal Properties: Helps digestion and assimilation. Combine with cascara sagrada for relief of constipation. Helps purify blood, activate the liver and build reproductive organs.

How to Use: Fresh or dried berries brewed into tea or extract, as directed.

Cautions: Do not take if pregnant.

Papaya

Tropical fruit with enzyme action.

Parts Used: Pulp of fruit.

Medicinal Properties: Contains papain, an enzyme that helps digest protein. Good for indigestion.

How to Use: Tablets or juice, as directed.

Cautions: None known.

Parsley

Popular garden herb, rich in vitamin B and potassium, used as garnish on plates, and can be eaten.

Parts Used: Leaves, seeds and roots.

Medicinal Properties: A good diuretic, excellent for gallbladder problems, including gall stones. Also good for bedwetting, edema, goiter, indigestion and gas, and menstrual problems.

How to Use: Eat raw, or make into tea. Tablets, as directed.

Cautions: Juice or oil may be too potent for pregnant women.

Passion Flower

Considered a safe natural alternative to sleeping pills.

Parts Used: Plant and flower.

Medicinal Properties: "Nature's tranquilizer" may relieve nervousness and its symptoms, and muscle spasms.

How to Use: Extract, as directed.

Cautions: May cause drowsiness in some people. Do not take during pregnancy or if driving.

Pau D'Arco

An Inca herb. This tree from the rain forests of Brazil is now being seriously researched for its anti-cancer properties.

Parts Used: Inner bark

Medicinal Properties: An immune booster with anti-tumor, anti-virus and anti-fungal abilities. Good for anemia, asthma, candida, colitis and psoriasis.

How to Use: Capsules, extract or tea, as directed. Look for products that use the only purple flower variety.

Cautions: None known.

Pennyroyal

Native Americans used this herb to relieve menstrual cramps.

Parts Used: Whole plant

Medicinal Properties: This blood purifier and diuretic induces sweating, promotes menstruation, helps heal colds, coughs and gas.

How to Use: Extract or dried herb, as directed.

Cautions: Do not use if pregnant (may induce abortion and hemorrhaging). Overdose may cause kidney and liver damage. Used on advice of licensed practitioner.

Peppermint

A common garden herb full of healing powers, mistakenly used only as a garnish.

Parts Used: Leaves and stems.

Medicinal Properties: Helps break down fats in heavy rich food and increases breast milk production. Aids colic, diarrhea, headaches, indigestion, menstrual cramps, kidney and urinary tract infections, colds, fevers, flu and nausea. May be helpful during a difficult labor.

How to Use: Internally, oil extract, as directed or herb, fresh or dried, as tea, as directed.

Cautions: None known.

Plantain

North American settlers brought this herb from Europe and introduced it the the Native Americans. Both cultures benefited from this useful and common broad-leaf weed.

Parts Used: Whole plant

Medicinal Properties: Effective for kidney and bladder ailments. Good for lymphatic system. Helps builds tissue. When used externally, helps ulcerated skin, insect bites and burns.

How to Use: Internally, capsules or herb, as directed. Externally, extract, as directed.

Cautions: None known.

Pleurisy Root

Used by Native Americans, this is now a common herb for bronchial problems.

Parts Used: Root

Medicinal Properties: Good for lungs and respiratory system, and as a digestive aid.

How to Use: Extract or dried herb, as directed.

Cautions: Use only reputable commercial preparations as fresh root may be dangerous.

Psyllium

This gentle, effective fiber food is now added to some commerical dry cereals.

Parts Used: Seeds

Medicinal Properties: Good for colon cleansing, constipation, hemorrhoids and gastro-intestinal irritations. May help prevent heart disease.

How to Use: Ground seeds or powder. Mix 1/2 teaspoon in 1 cup liquid. Build up to 1 teaspoon, three times a day when body becomes accustomed to it.

Cautions: Always drink lots of liquids with this herb.

Raspberry Leaves

Early settlers used the leaves, and especially the stems, for a refreshing tea when regular tea was unavailable.

Parts Used: Leaves and stems.

Medicinal Properties: Alleviates sore throats, fever blisters and menstrual cramps. May help shorten delivery by preparing uterus for childbirth.

How to Use: Extract or dried herb, as directed.

Cautions: Do not use during early pregnancy, and only in last two months under direction of licensed practitioner.

Red Clover

Red clover came to North America English settlers, and in the absence of medical doctors, this native plant of the British Isles served as a useful medicine.

Parts Used: Blossoms and leaves.

Medicinal Properties: A rich source of silica and other minerals, it has a relaxing and blood purifying benefits. Good for overall health, skin and lung inflammation, gout, arthritis, tuberculosis, whooping cough and fighting bacteria. May help fight cancerous growths.

How to Use: Extract or capsules, as directed.

Cautions: Consult qualified practitioner in treating cancer.

Rosehips

The shiny orange-red berries on wild and domestic rose bushes have a rich vitamin C content.

Parts Used: Seeds and pods.

Medicinal Properties: Excellent source of vitamin C, so it is effective against colds, coughs, diarrhea, scurvy and stress.

How to Use: Dry powder or capsules, as directed.

Cautions: None known.

Rosemary

A popular kitchen herb found growing on tough evergreen shrubs.

Parts Used: Leaves and stems.

Medicinal Properties: Good for dizziness from ear disturbances, headaches and migraines and sharpening memory. A good rinse for hair, stimulates hair growth and rids scalp of dandruff.

How to Use: Dried herb as tea or essential oil, as directed.

Cautions: None known.

Sage

A popular kitchen herb associated with longevity.

Parts Used: Leaves

Medicinal Properties: Aids in reducing night sweats typical of tuberculosis. Mouthwash for sore gums. Tea for stomach cramps and gas. Good for digestion, stopping flow of milk in nursing mother and nervous conditions.

How to Use: Powder or dry herb for tea, as directed.

Cautions: None known.

Sarsaparilla

Often used in beverages, this useful herb came to North America with the Spanish settlers.

Parts Used: Root

Medicinal Properties: A natural steroid. Increases energy, eliminates poisons from the blood and helps clean the system of infections. Clears skin ailments such as eczema and psoriasis. Also good for arthritis, colds, catarrh and gout.

How to Use: Extract or capsules, as directed.

Cautions: None known.

Saw Palmetto

Found in the Southeast coast of the US. Settlers learned of its beneficial qualities from watching animals lean over fences to eat the berries.

Parts Used: Berries

Medicinal Properties: Helps maintain proper urinary function in mature men. Soothing to reproductive organs and may help excessive urination from enlarged prostate. Good for coughs and colds, asthma, arthritis and bronchitis.

How to Use: Extract, as directed.

Cautions: Always consult physician if suffering painful urination, bleeding or enlarged prostate.

Senna

This powerful herb is almost always used combined with other herbs, especially ones that aid digestion.

Parts Used: Leaves

Medicinal Properties: A powerful stimulant and laxative that should be combined with ginger or fennel to relieve constipation and prevent cramps.

How to Use: Internally, take dry herb or tablets, only as directed. Externally, paste for skin irritations.

Cautions: Do not use during pregnancy or if you have an inflamed intestinal tract. Use on advice of licensed practitioner.

Shepherd's Purse

Another name for this herb is "mothers' hearts."

Parts Used: Whole plant

Medicinal Properties: A diuretic and astringent good for dysentery,

rheumatism and catarrh. Also helps control any hemorrhaging of kidneys, lungs, stomach and uterus. Beneficial for hemorrhaging after childbirth and during menstruation.

How to Use: Dry herb as tea or capsules, as directed.

Cautions: Do not use if pregnant.

Shiitake Mushroom

A popular food item with immune boosting abilities.

Parts Used: Tops

Medicinal Properties: Lowers blood cholesterol. Seems to help in reduction of tumors and enhance the body's natural defenses. May be helpful for people suffering from clinical depression.

How to Use: Capsules, as directed or eat dry or fresh mushrooms.

Cautions: Consult with licensed practitioner, but small amounts are quite safe.

Skullcap

Also known as "mad dog weed", this plant is named for its cap-shaped flower, and was a traditional remedy for rabies.

Parts Used: Whole herb

Medicinal Properties: Helps menstrual cramps and muscle pain, alcoholism and high blood pressure. Good for neuralgia, aches and pains, rheumatism, nervous tension and insomnia.

How to Use: Capsules, dried herb or extract, as directed.

Cautions: None known.

Slippery Elm

A gentle and effective remedy popular with early settlers.

Parts Used: Inner bark, fresh or dried.

Medicinal Properties: Soothing to throat, esophagus and ulcerated or cancerous stomach. Both strengthening and healing, it is good for inflammation of bladder and kidney, bowels, heart, stomach and female organs.

How to Use: Tablets or lozenges, as directed.

Cautions: None known.

Squaw Vine

A long used folk remedy to help the body prepare for childbirth.

Parts Used: Root

Medicinal Properties: Good for female organs. Used by women six weeks before delivery to aid childbirth. Helps menstrual cramps, insomnia and urinary ailments.

How to Use: Dried herb or tablets, as directed.

Cautions: Licensed practitioner will tell you optimal dosage for female problems.

St. John's Wort

Popular in Europe in the Middle Ages, this herb was often consumed to ward off evil spirits.

Parts Used: Tops and flowers.

Medicinal Properties: Calming and good for anxiety, it helps with cramps and irregular menstruation, fights viral infection and promotes healing of skin wounds.

How to Use: Internally, extract, as directed.

Cautions: This herb can cause sensitivity to light, so avoid sun exposure.

Suma

This herb from the tropical rain forests of Brazil was found by the natives to have medicinal qualities. Works similar to ginseng.

Parts Used: Root

Medicinal Properties: Good for chronic fatigue and as an energy tonic when recovering from illness.

How to Use: Capsules or tablets, as directed.

Cautions: None known.

Tea Tree

A tiny bottle of this effective antiseptic is wise to bring on wilderness trips for cuts and bruises.

Parts Used: Leaves

Medicinal Properties: An effective germicide and fungicide, used in treatment of wounds and infections. Also good for athlete's foot, cold sores, cystitis and dermatitis.

How to Use: Externally, oil, as directed.

Cautions: None known.

Thyme

This medicinal wonder is easily grown in any garden or patio pot.

Parts Used: Whole plant

Medicinal Properties: Helps relieve nervous disorders, fevers and headaches. Lowers cholesterol, helps sinusitis, clears mucus and aids asthma and chronic respiratory problems. Good for athlete's foot.

How to Use: Dried herb, made into tea or gargle. Extract, rub between toes daily for athlete's foot.

Cautions: None known.

Turmeric

The bright yellow spice in curry.

Parts Used: Root or rhizome.

Medicinal Properties: Protects gallbladder, helps arthritis, helps prevent blood clots, relieves arthritis and is beneficial to digestion.

How to Use: Capsules, as directed or a spice in cooking.

Cautions: None known.

Uva Ursi

This diuretic is also known as bearberry.

Parts Used: Leaves

Medicinal Properties: Good for diabetes, relieving pain of cystitis and nephritis and hemorrhoids. A good toning agent for most internal organs.

How to Use: Capsules or dried herb, as directed.

Cautions: None known.

Valerian

This effective, non-addictive tranquilizer is commonly available in Russian drug stores to help people cope with stress.

Parts Used: Root and rhizome.

Medicinal Properties: Good for soothing nerves without a narcotic effect. Promotes sleep, relieves gas pains and stomach cramps, helps

with heart palpitations and epileptic fits and is good for children with measles and scarlet fever.

How to Use: Extract, capsules or tablets, as directed.

Cautions: High doses may cause paralysis and weakening of heartbeat, so seek professional advice.

Water Cress

A pungent, peppery green plant sold in bunches in most markets.

Parts Used: Leaves, flowers and roots.

Medicinal Properties: Helps body use oxygen and stimulates metabolism increasing physical endurance. Good for bladder, kidney and liver problems and may dissolve kidney stones.

How to Use: Dried or fresh herb, extract or tablets, as directed.

Cautions: None known.

White Willow

This bark extract was used for headahces long before aspirin was manufactured. Early settlers used it in much the same way as aspirin is used today.

Parts Used: Bark

Medicinal Properties: Natural anti-inflammatory and pain reliever, lowers fevers, helps relieve arthritis, bursitis, dandruff, eye problems, eczema, flu and chills, headaches, nosebleeds and rheumatism.

How to Use: Tablets or concentrated extract, as directed.

Cautions: None known.

Wild Yam

A natural source for production of progesterone.

Parts Used: Root

Medicinal Properties: Cream used for menopausal symptoms. Relieves nausea due to pregnancy. Good for acne, angina, diarrhea, dysentery, and gallbladder and liver disorders.

How to Use: Internally, tablets or extract, as directed. Externally, cream, as directed.

Cautions: None known.

Wintergreen

As one of the mint family, this plant has many of the same properties, but with its own distinctive flavor.

Parts Used: Whole plant

Medicinal Properties: Famous for relieving pain of rheumatism, gas and headaches. Good for neuralgia and urinary problems.

How to Use: Extract, as directed.

Cautions: None known.

Witch Hazel

An old remedy, this clear astringent is available for insect bites, oily skin and other conditions.

Parts Used: Bark and leaves.

Medicinal Properties: Effective anti-inflammatory. Soothing for bruises and minor cuts. Slows internal bleeding and reduces pain of dysentery, diarrhea and hemorrhoids. Clears excess oil on skin.

How to Use: Externally, extract as directed.

Cautions: None known.

Wood Betony

Rarely used now, this herb has had a long history of healing ailments.

Parts Used: Leaves

Medicinal Properties: Good for stomach cramps, gout, headaches, colic, colds and indigestion. May be effective for jaundice, tuberculosis and Parkinson's disease. Good for the heart.

How to Use: Extract or capsules, as directed.

Cautions: Avoid during pregnancy.

Wormwood

An extremely bitter tasting plant.

Parts Used: Tops and leaves.

Medicinal Properties: Helps to relieve female complaints, diabetes and diarrhea.

How to Use: Used as a tea, in combination with other herbs.

Cautions: This herb is quite powerful. Seek advice of a herbalist.

Yarrow

Otherwise known as nosebleed and millefoil.

Parts Used: Whole herb

Medicinal Properties: Good for colds and flu. High in tannic acid, so helps stop bleeding. Good to stimulate production of fresh blood cells in bone marrow, relieve diarrhea, dysentery and female problems. Soothes nerves and heart.

How to Use: Typically used as tea, often in combination with other herbs.

Cautions: None known.

Yellow Dock

An plain-looking weed that has unique tonic qualities.

Parts Used: Leaves and roots.

Medicinal Properties: Rich in minerals, especially iron. A laxative and blood purifier. It restores lymphatic system and helps skin problems.

How to Use: Internally, capsules or tea, as directed. Externally, ointments, as directed.

Cautions: None known.

Yucca

A common succulent desert plant with some flowering and decorative varieties.

Parts Used: Root

Medicinal Properties: Has steroid saponins which are good for arthritis and rheumatism.

How to Use: Capsules, tablets or extract, as directed.

Cautions: Long term use may interfere with fat soluble vitamins.

Guide to Herbal Combinations

Sometimes a combination of different herbs and vitamins work synergistically to either treat existing problems, or help maintain good health. Over the centuries, herbal practitioners have tested and experimented with different herbs, alone and in combination, and modern herbalists have brought us some effective combination formulas.

It is always a good idea to consult a licensed practitioner when using herbs alone, or in combination, and there are many good sources you can read to become more knowledgeable. (See Recommended Reading section.) But, the best indication is your own experience. Since we are each unique, when you find a formula that works, treasure it. Use each herb combination as directed.

Anxiety

Herb Combination: Valerian, passion flower, wood betony, black cohosh, skullcap, hops and ginger. Helps anxiety and irritability.

Colds and Flu

Herb Combination: Goldenseal, cayenne and bayberry. Also good for sore throat and upper respiratory congestion.

Depressed Immunity

Herb Combination: Astragalus, feverfew, ginkgo, St. John's wort and suma. Works as natural antibiotic and tonic for the immune system. Tones the nerves, stomach, heart and circulatory system.

Dieting Aid

Herb Combination: Chickweed, safflower, burdock, parsley, kelp, papaya, licorice, fennel, echinacea, black walnut and hawthorn. Enhances a diet program by aiding metabolism and elimination.

Digestive Problems

Herb Combination: Papaya, peppermint, ginger, catnip, fennel and saw palmetto. Good for irritable bowel and intestinal irritation.

Energy Booster

Herb Combination: Siberian ginseng, cayenne, kelp, peppermint, ginger and gotu kola.

Fevers

Herb Combination: Echinacea, goldenseal, comfrey, myrrh, blue vervain, garlic and kelp. Helps fight infections.

Heart Disease

Herb Combination: Hawthorn, pectin, black cohosh and cayenne. Works by reducing cholesterol and helps lower triglycerides in blood.

Impaired Circulation

Herb Combination: Cayenne, ginger, kelp, gentian root and blue ver-vain. Helps cold hands and feet, varicose veins, nausea and colds.

Liver and Bowel Problems

Herb Combination: Dandelion, cascara sagrada, licorice, celery seed, cayenne and wild yam. Helps regulate elimination process.

Memory Problems and Senility

Herb Combination: Gotu kola, Siberian ginseng, peppermint, skullcap, wood betony and kelp. Increases circulation which aids body functions.

Overeating

Herb Combination: Pectin, guar gum, psyllium, kava kava and ephedra. Works as appetite suppressant.

Respiratory Problems

Herb Combination: Pleurisy root, slippery elm, mullein, chickweed, horehound, licorice, comfrey, kelp, cayenne and saw palmetto. Soothes smokers' cough and relieves inflamed and irritated lungs.

Water Retention

Herb Combination: Cornsilk, uva ursi, parsley, buchu, juniper berries, kelp and cayenne. Helps rid body of excess water.

Part 3

Common Ailments

Acne

Herbs: Burdock, chaparral, chlorophyll, echinacea, garlic, gotu kola, red clover and yellow dock.

Vitamins: A, B-complex, B3, B6, C, E and F.

Minerals: Potassium and sulfur.

AIDS

(Acquired Immune Deficiency Syndrome)

Herbs: Cayenne, Korean ginseng, garlic, milk thistle, pau d'arco, shiitake mushroom, suma and yucca.

Vitamins: A, B6, B12, B-complex and E.

Minerals: High potency multi-mineral formulas, plus zinc and copper.

Alcoholism

Herbs: Cayenne, dandelion, Siberian ginseng, goldenseal, licorice root, lobelia, nettle, skullcap and valerian.

Vitamins: A, B-complex, C, D and E.

Minerals: Zinc and magnesium.

Allergies

Herbs: Burdock root, cayenne, chaparral, eyebright, lobelia, goldenseal and nettle.

Vitamins: A, B-complex, B3, B5, B6, B12, C, E and F.

Minerals: Calcium, magnesium and manganese.

Anemia

Herbs: Dandelion, fenugreek, kelp and yellow dock.

Vitamins: Complete multi-vitamin with additional C.

Minerals: Complete multi-mineral with added iron.

Arteriosclerosis

Herbs: Cayenne, evening primrose oil, garlic, goldenseal and rosehips.

Vitamins: B-complex, B3, C, E, inositol and choline.

Minerals: Calcium and magnesium.

Arthritis

Herbs: Alfalfa, black cohosh, burdock, chaparral, devil's claw and yucca.

Vitamins: B-complex, B3, C, D, E, F and P.

Minerals: Good multi-mineral supplement.

Asthma

Herbs: Lobelia, fenugreek, mullein and nettle.

Vitamins: A, B-complex, B2, B3, B5, B6, B12, C, E, F and PABA.

Minerals: Manganese

Athlete's Foot

Herbs: Calendula

Vitamins: Apply vitamin C crystals.

Athletic Injuries

Herbs: Arnica, white willow, comfrey, black walnut, lobelia and skullcap.

Vitamins: Good multi-vitamin.

Minerals: Good multi-mineral.

Bad Breath

Herbs: Myrrh, parsley, peppermint and rosemary.

Vitamins: A, B-complex, B3, B6, C and PABA.

Minerals: Magnesium and zinc.

Baldness

Herbs: Aloe vera, kelp, rosemary, nettle, yarrow and yucca.

Vitamins: A, B-complex, B3, B5, B6, C, biotin, folic acid and inositol.

Minerals: Copper, iodine, selenium and magnesium.

Bee Stings

Herbs: Echinacea, pau d'arco and yellow dock.

Vitamins: B1 is a repellent or C, if stung, to ease allergic reaction.

Minerals: Calcium

Blood Cleanser

Herbs: Red clover, chaparral, dandelion, garlic and burdock.

Minerals: Iron

Blood Clots

Herbs: Comfrey, garlic, goldenseal, kelp and evening primrose.

Vitamins: B-complex, B3, C, E, inositol and choline.

Minerals: Calcium, magnesium and selenium.

Blood Pressure (High)

Herbs: Cayenne, garlic, hawthorn, kelp, valerian and yarrow.

Vitamins: A, B-complex, B3, B5, C, D, E, P, inositol and choline.

Minerals: Calcium, magnesium and potassium.

Blood Pressure (Low)

Herbs: Garlic, hawthorn, Siberian ginseng, kelp, goldenseal and ginger.

Vitamins: A, B-complex, B5, C, E and P.

Blood Purifier

Herbs: Alfalfa, burdock, chaparral, echinacea, devil's claw, Oregon grape, pau d'arco, red clover and yellow dock.

Minerals: Iron and germanium.

Boils

Herbs: Chaparral, dandelion, echinacea, lobelia, mullein and clover.

Vitamins: A, C and E.

Minerals: Zinc, as a preventative.

Bowel Cleanser

Herbs: Cascara sagrada, goldenseal, lobelia, psyllium seeds, licorice, red raspberry and senna.

Vitamins: B-complex

Breastfeeding

Herbs: Alfalfa, blessed thistle, fennel, raspberry and marshmallow. Sage will help dry up milk when ready to wean.

Vitamins: Extra C, if baby has a cold.

Breathing Problems

Herbs: Lobelia, marshmallow root and mullein.

Vitamins: C

Bright's Disease

Herbs: Alfalfa, bayberry, catnip, dandelion, fennel, ginger, horsetail and wild yam.

Vitamins: A, B-complex, C, D, E and choline.

Bronchitis

Herbs: Eucalyptus, lobelia, chickweed and slippery elm. Cayenne with ginger clears the lungs.

Vitamins: A, B12, C and E.

Minerals: A good multi-mineral plus zinc.

Burns

Herbs: Aloe vera and comfrey.

Vitamins: C, E and PABA. (Apply E oil and aloe vera to burn.)

Minerals: Zinc

Bursitis

Herbs: Alfalfa, chaparral and comfrey. Mullein as poultice externally.

Vitamins: A, B12, B-complex, C, E and P.

Minerals: Calcium and magnesium.

Cancer

(Be sure to seek professional advice.)

Herbs: Burdock, chaparral, garlic, ginger, ginseng, goldenseal, echinacea, pau d'arco, red clover, suma and yucca.

Vitamins: A, B3, B-complex, C and E.

Minerals: Germanium, magnesium, potassium and selenium.

Candida Albicans

Herbs: Black walnut, garlic and pau d'arco.

Vitamins: Biotin

Canker Sores

Herbs: Burdock root, goldenseal and pau d'arco.

Vitamins: A, B5, B12, B-complex and large doses of C.

Minerals: Iron

Carpal Tunnel Syndrome

Herbs: Ginger

Vitamins: B-complex, B6 and C.

Minerals: Calcium and magnesium.

Cataracts

Herbs: Eyebright and bilberry.

Vitamins: B2

Minerals: Copper, magnesium, selenium and zinc.

Chicken Pox

Herbs: Cayenne, chickweed, echinacea, lobelia and red clover.

Vitamins: A multi-vitamin plus extra A, C and E.

Minerals: Potassium and zinc.

Chronic Fatigue

Herbs: Astragalus, cayenne, echinacea, Siberian ginseng, Korean ginseng, gotu kola, lobelia, alfalfa and garlic.

Vitamins: A, C with bioflavonoids, B-complex (high potency), E, D and folic acid.

Minerals: Iron, magnesium, manganese, potassium, selenium and zinc.

Circulation

Herbs: Cayenne, black cohosh, bayberry, butcher's broom, ginkgo and yarrow.

Vitamins: A, B3, C and E.

Minerals: Calcium, magnesium and potassium.

Cirrhosis
(of the Liver)

Herbs: Barberry, burdock, dandelion, echinacea, fennel, garlic, goldenseal, hops, milk thistle, red clover and suma.

Vitamins: A, B3, B12, B-complex, C, D, E and K.

Minerals: Magnesium and zinc.

Cold Feet

Herbs: Cayenne, bayberry and kelp.

Vitamins: Vitamin E and B3.

Minerals: A good multi-mineral.

Cold Sores

Vitamins: Vitamin C and E oil, applied on affected part.

Minerals: Zinc. The amino acid, lysine is good as well.

Colds and Flu

Herbs: Echinacea, cayenne, red clover, raspberry tea, chaparral, rosehips, garlic and goldenseal.

Vitamins: A, B6 and C.

Minerals: A good multi-mineral.

Colic

Herbs: Catnip, fennel, chamomile and peppermint.

Colitis

Herbs: Alfalfa, bayberry, chamomile, caraway, garlic, peppermint, plantain, valerian and wild yam.

Vitamins: A, B6, B-complex, C and E.

Minerals: Calcium lactate, iron, magnesium and potassium.

Constipation

Herbs: Aloe vera, cascara sagrada, psyllium, damiana and senna.

Vitamins: A, B-complex, C, D and E.

Minerals: Calcium, magnesium, potassium and zinc.

Coughs

Herbs: Cayenne, fenugreek, goldenseal, lungwort and mullein.

Vitamins: A, B6, C and P.

Crohn's Disease

Herbs: Echinacea, garlic, goldenseal, pau d'arco and rosehips.

Vitamins: A, B12, B-complex and E.

Minerals: A good multi-mineral.

Croup

Herbs: Echinacea, fenugreek and goldenseal.

Vitamins: A, C and E.

Minerals: Zinc

Cystitis

Herbs: Cranberry, alfalfa and uva ursi.

Vitamins: A, B-complex, D, E and choline.

Minerals: Calcium, magnesium and potassium.

Dandruff

Herbs: Burdock, chaparral, red clover, nettle and yarrow (made into tea and applied to scalp).

Vitamins: A, B-complex, B6, C and E.

Minerals: Selenium and zinc.

Depression

Herbs: Cayenne, damiana, gotu kola, St. John's wort, skullcap, Siberian ginseng and yucca.

Vitamins: B3, B6, B12, B-complex and large doses of vitamin C.

Minerals: Calcium, magnesium and zinc, plus good multi-mineral.

Dermatitis

Herbs: Aloe vera (externally), burdock, dandelion, evening primrose, garlic, goldenseal, pau d'arco and yellow dock.

Vitamins: A, B-complex, B2, B3, B6, D, E and biotin.

Minerals: Sulfur, in ointment form, zinc and potassium.

Diabetes

Herbs: Cayenne, licorice root, mullein, suma, juniper and uva ursi.

Vitamins: A, B-complex, B1, B2, B6, B12, C, E, choline and inositol.

Minerals: Calcium, chromium, iron, potassium, magnesium and zinc.

Diarrhea

Herbs: Raspberry, slippery elm and yucca.

Vitamins: A, B-complex, B1, B2, B3, B6, C, folic acid and choline.

Minerals: Calcium, chlorine, iron, magnesium, potassium and sodium.

Digestive Problems

Herbs: Aloe vera, chamomile, cayenne, fennel, ginger, goldenseal, licorice, marshmallow and papaya.

Vitamins: A, B3, B-complex and biotin.

Minerals: Calcium, copper, iodine, phosphorus, potassium and zinc.

Drug Addictions

Herbs: Pau d'arco, chamomile, licorice root and lobelia.

Vitamins: B-complex and C.

Minerals: Calcium and potassium.

Ear Infections

Herbs: Blue cohosh, echinacea, garlic, mullein oil, skullcap and St. John's wort.

Vitamins: A, B-complex and C.

Minerals: Calcium and zinc.

Eczema

Herbs: Aloe vera, chickweed, evening primrose oil, pau d'arco, red clover, milk thistle and yellow dock.

Vitamins: A, B-complex, C, D, PABA, biotin, choline and inositol.

Minerals: Magnesium, sulfur ointment and zinc ointment.

Edema

Herbs: Buchu, dandelion, juniper, parsley, uva ursi and yarrow.

Vitamins: B1, B6, B-complex, C, D and E.

Minerals: Calcium, copper and potassium.

Emphysema

Herbs: Anise seed oil, garlic, lobelia and mullein.

Vitamins: A, B-complex, C, D, E and folic acid.

Epilepsy

Herbs: Black cohosh, nettle, hyssop, Irish moss and skullcap.

Vitamins: A, B-complex, niacin, B6, C, D and E.

Minerals: Calcium, chromium, iron and magnesium.

Eye Problems

Herbs: Eyebright and bilberry.

Vitamins: A, B1, B2, B3, B6, C, D and E.

Minerals: Calcium, copper, manganese, selenium, magnesium and zinc.

Fevers and Flu

Herbs: Echinacea at onset, feverfew, blessed thistle, calendula, bayberry, ephedra, eucalyptus oil, cayenne, fenugreek, goldenseal, lungwort and mullein.

Vitamins: A, B-complex, B3, C and E.

Minerals: Calcium, phosphorus, potassium and sodium.

Food Poisoning

Herbs: Pau d'arco

Vitamins: C and E.

Minerals: A good multi-mineral.

Gas

Herbs: Catnip, ginger, peppermint and horseradish.

Vitamins: B-complex

Glaucoma

Herbs: Eyebright and bilberry.

Vitamins: A, B2, B-complex, C, D and E.

Minerals: A good multi-mineral.

Goiter

Herbs: Kelp

Vitamins: A, B6, B-complex, choline, C and E.

Minerals: Calcium and iodine.

Gout

Herbs: Burdock, dandelion, lobelia, nettle, pau d'arco and yucca.

Vitamins: A, B-complex, C and E.

Minerals: Calcium, magnesium and potassium.

Hay Fever

Herbs: Echinacea, nettle, eyebright, goldenseal and yarrow.

Vitamins: A, B-complex, C with bioflavonoids and E.

Headache

Herbs: Chamomile and feverfew.

Vitamins: A, B-complex, C, D and E.

Minerals: Calcium, magnesium, potassium and zinc.

Heart Attack

Herbs: Cayenne, comfrey, evening primrose oil, garlic, goldenseal and rosehips.

Vitamins: B-complex, C, E, niacin, inositol and choline.

Minerals: Calcium and magnesium.

Heart Burn

Herbs: Chamomile, papaya (chewable) and marshmallow.

Hemorrhoids

Herbs: Butcher's broom, witch hazel, slippery elm, goldenseal, lobelia, mullein, psyllium husks and yellow dock.

Vitamins: A, B-complex, C, E and E oil topically.

Minerals: Multi-mineral plus calcium.

Hiatus Hernia

Herbs: Aloe vera juice, goldenseal and red clover.

Vitamins: A, B-complex and C.

Minerals: A multi-mineral plus zinc.

Hyperactivity

Herbs: Evening primrose oil, lobelia, skullcap, St. John's wort, valerian and ginkgo.

Vitamins: High potency B vitamins and C.

Minerals: Good multi-mineral, in high doses.

Hyperthyroidism

Herbs: Alfalfa, calendula, echinacea, goldenseal, lobelia, mullein, saw palmetto and skullcap.

Vitamins: A, B-complex, C and E.

Minerals: Calcium, magnesium and potassium.

Hypoglycemia

Herbs: Some people with hypoglycemia cannot tolerate goldenseal, as it lowers blood sugar.

Vitamins: A, B-complex, C, E and folic acid.

Minerals: Magnesium and potassium.

Hypothyroidism

Vitamins: A, B1, C, D and E.

Minerals: Calcium, magnesium and potassium.

Immune Deficiency

Herbs: Echinacea, chaparral, Korean ginseng, pau d'arco, rosemary and goldenseal.

Vitamins: A good multi-vitamin plus extra B6, B12, C and E.

Minerals: A good multi-mineral, preferably time-released.

Impotence

Herbs: Damiana
Vitamins: E, PABA and folic acid.
Minerals: Zinc, iodine and calcium.

Infertility

Herbs: Dong quai and gotu kola.
Vitamins: A, B6, B-complex and E.
Minerals: A good multi-mineral.

Insomnia

Herbs: Catnip, hops, skullcap, pau d'arco and valerian.
Vitamins: B-complex, D and E.
Minerals: Calcium, iron, magnesium and potassium.

Jet Lag

Herbs: Gotu kola and Korean ginseng.
Vitamins: B-complex and a multi-vitamin with extra C and E.
Minerals: A good multi-mineral.

Kidney Functions

Herbs: Garlic, parsley and cranberry juice.

Kidney Stones

Herbs: Cornsilk, dandelion, juniper, parsley, thyme and uva ursi.
Vitamins: A, B-complex, C, E and choline.
Minerals: Magnesium and potassium.

Leg Cramps

Herbs: Comfrey, horsetail and skullcap.

Vitamins: B-complex, C, D and E.
Minerals: Calcium, magnesium and phosphorus.

Leg Ulcers

Herbs: Cayenne, bayberry, butcher's broom, ginkgo and yarrow.
Vitamins: A, B3, B12, C and E.
Minerals: Calcium, iron, magnesium and potassium.

Leukemia

(Be sure to seek professional advice.)
Herbs: Pau d'arco and nettle.
Vitamins: B-complex, added B12, C and E.
Minerals: Copper, iron and zinc.

Liver Disorders

Herbs: Dandelion and horsetail.
Vitamins: A, B-complex, C, E and choline.

Melanoma

(Be sure to seek professional advice.)
Herbs: Kelp and pau d'arco.
Vitamins: A, B-complex, with added B12, niacin, folic acid, C and E.
Minerals: A good multi-mineral plus added calcium and magnesium.

Memory Problems

Herbs: Cayenne, ginkgo, gotu kola, Korean ginseng and lobelia.
Vitamins: Choline
Minerals: A good multi-mineral.

Meningitis

(Be sure to seek professional advice.)
Herbs: Catnip and garlic.

Vitamins: A good multi-vitamin plus extra A, C and D.

Minerals: A good high-potency mineral, plus extra calcium, zinc and germanium.

Menopause

Herbs: Black cohosh, blessed thistle, dong quai, licorice, sarsaparilla and Siberian ginseng.

Vitamins: A, B-complex, C, D and E.

Minerals: Calcium, magnesium, potassium and selenium.

Menstrual Problems

(Be sure to seek professional advice, especially if on the birth control pill or taking hormone replacement.)

Herbs: Blessed thistle, calendula, dong quai, red raspberry, pennyroyal, uva ursi, valerian, white willow and chamomile.

Vitamins: B-complex, C and E.

Minerals: Calcium and iodine.

Migraine Headaches

Herbs: Chamomile and feverfew.

Vitamins: B-complex, B3, C and PABA.

Minerals: Calcium, magnesium and potassium.

Mononucleosis

Vitamins: A, B-complex, C, biotin and choline.

Minerals: Potassium

Morning Sickness

Herbs: Red raspberry, peppermint, alfalfa, catnip and ginger.

Vitamins: A good multi-vitamin plus B6, C and K.

Motion Sickness

Herbs: Ginkgo and ginger.

Vitamins: B-complex plus B6.

Minerals: Charcoal tablets

Mouth Sores

Herbs: Aloe vera, goldenseal, myrrh and red raspberry.

Vitamins: A, B-complex, C and E.

Minerals: Iron, magnesium, phosphorus and zinc.

Multiple Sclerosis

Herbs: Evening primrose oil, kelp, skullcap and St. John's wort.

Vitamins: B-complex, C, E and inositol.

Minerals: Calcium, copper, iron, magnesium, manganese, selenium and zinc.

Mumps

Herbs: Bayberry, echinacea, ginger, lobelia and mullein.

Vitamins: A, B-complex, C and E.

Minerals: A good multi-mineral.

Muscular Dystrophy

Herbs: Saw palmetto

Vitamins: A, B-complex, C, E and choline.

Minerals: Potassium

Nausea

Herbs: Cayenne, chaparral, garlic, ginger, raspberry, red clover, rosehips and goldenseal.

Vitamins: A, B6 and C.

Minerals: Magnesium

Nervous Problems

Herbs: Evening primrose oil, hops, skullcap and valerian.

Vitamins: B-complex and C.

Minerals: Calcium, iodine, iron, magnesium, phosphorus, potassium, silicon and sodium.

Neuritis

Herbs: Black cohosh, lobelia, skullcap, and valerian.

Vitamins: B-complex

Minerals: A good multi-mineral plus extra calcium and magnesium.

Night Blindness

Herbs: Bilberry and eyebright.

Vitamins: A good multi-vitamin.

Minerals: Calcium, copper, manganese, magnesium, potassium, selenium and zinc.

Obesity

Herbs: Chickweed, hawthorn, kelp, licorice and papaya leaves.

Vitamins: B-complex, C, E, choline, folic acid and inositol.

Minerals: Chromium

Osteoarthritis

Herbs: Alfalfa, black cohosh, burdock, cayenne, chaparral, devil's claw, valerian and yucca.

Vitamins: B-complex, C, D and E.

Minerals: A good multi-mineral plus calcium and magnesium.

Osteoporosis

Herbs: Feverfew and horsetail.

Vitamins: B12, C, D and E.

Minerals: Calcium, copper, fluoride, magnesium and phosphorus.

Parkinson's Disease

Herbs: Ginseng, damiana and cayenne.

Vitamins: B-complex, B2, B6, C and E.

Minerals: Calcium and magnesium.

Phlebitis

Herbs: Ginkgo, horse chestnut and yarrow.

Vitamins: B-complex, C and E.

Minerals: A good multi-mineral.

Pneumonia

(Be sure to seek professional advice.)

Herbs: Comfrey, echinacea, eucalyptus, fenugreek, licorice and mullein.

Vitamins: A, B-complex, C with bioflavonoids, E and K.

Minerals: Zinc

Pre-Natal Preparation

Herbs: Blessed thistle, chamomile, lobelia and red raspberry.

Vitamins: A, B-complex, C, D and E.

Minerals: A good multi-mineral plus extra calcium, magnesium and phosphorus.

Psoriasis

Herbs: Chickweed, dandelion,

goldenseal, lobelia, skullcap, St. John's wort and yellow dock.

Vitamins: A, B-complex, C, D, E and folic acid.

Minerals: Calcium, magnesium, sulfur and zinc ointment.

Rheumatic Fever

Herbs: Catnip, dandelion, fenugreek, garlic, lobelia, thyme and pau d'arco.

Vitamins: A good multi-vitamin plus extra A, B2, B6, C, D and E.

Minerals: Zinc

Rheumatism

Herbs: Alfalfa, chaparral, cayenne, fennel, garlic, pau d'arco, red clover, red raspberry and yucca.

Vitamins: B-complex, C and E.

Minerals: Calcium, magnesium, phosphorus, potassium and zinc.

Sciatica

Herbs: Pau d'arco

Vitamins: B-complex, D and E.

Minerals: A good multi-mineral.

Senility

Herbs: Dandelion, ginkgo, ginseng, gotu kola, licorice and yellow dock.

Vitamins: A, B-complex, C and E.

Minerals: Zinc

Shingles

Herbs: Calendula

Vitamins: A, B-complex, and especially high doses of C and D.

Minerals: Calcium and magnesium.

Sinus Problems

Herbs: Comfrey, eyebright, fenugreek and goldenseal.

Vitamins: A, B-complex, C and E.

Minerals: Potassium and zinc.

Smoking

Herbs: Catnip, chaparral, hops, licorice, lobelia, skullcap, slippery elm and valerian.

Vitamins: A multi-vitamin with C.

Minerals: A multi-mineral.

Stress

Herbs: Black cohosh, cayenne, skullcap and valerian.

Vitamins: A, B-complex, C, D, E, PABA, folic acid and choline.

Minerals: Calcium, chromium, copper, iron, selenium and zinc.

Stroke

Herbs: Cayenne, comfrey, evening primrose oil, garlic, goldenseal and rosehips.

Vitamins: B-complex, B3, C, E, inositol and choline.

Minerals: A good multi-mineral plus calcium and magnesium.

Sunburn

Herbs: Aloe vera (externally)

Vitamins: B-complex, PABA, C and E.

Minerals: Calcium and zinc.

Teeth Grinding

Herbs: Chamomile, skullcap and valerian.

Vitamins: A good multi-vitamin, taken before bed.

Minerals: Calcium

Teething

Herbs: Lobelia, aloe vera gel or peppermint oil rubbed on gums.

Tinnitus
(Ringing in the Ears)

Herbs: Cayenne, black cohosh, bayberry, butcher's broom, ginkgo and yarrow.

Vitamins: A, B-complex, C and E.

Minerals: Calcium, magnesium, manganese and potassium.

Tonsillitis

Herbs: Bayberry, echinacea, ginger and pau d'arco.

Vitamins: A good multi-vitamin.

Minerals: A good multi-mineral.

Tumors
(Non-malignant)

Herbs: Dandelion, kelp, pau d'arco and red clover.

Vitamins: A, B-complex, C and E.

Minerals: A good multi-mineral.

Ulcers (Skin)

Herbs: Goldenseal and myrrh.

Vitamins: Folic acid, pantothenic acid, C and E.

Minerals: A good multi-mineral.

Ulcers (Stomach)

Herbs: Goldenseal, myrrh, pau d'arco,

red raspberry, slippery elm and valerian.

Vitamins: A, B-complex, C, D, E, choline and folic acid.

Minerals: Calcium, manganese and zinc.

Varicose Veins

Herbs: Butcher's broom, hawthorn, horse chestnut, witch hazel and yarrow.

Vitamins: B-complex, C and E.

Minerals: Potassium and zinc.

Warts

Herbs: Echinacea, garlic, goldenseal, onions and pau d'arco.

Vitamins: A, B-complex, C and E.

Minerals: Zinc

Water Retention

Herbs: Buchu, cranberry, dandelion, juniper, parsley and uva ursi.

Vitamins: B6 and C.

Minerals: Calcium and potassium.

Whooping Cough

Herbs: Horehound and valerian.

Vitamins: A, B-complex and C.

Minerals: Zinc

Yeast Infection

Herbs: Black walnut, garlic and pau d'arco.

Vitamins: A, C, E and biotin.

Recommended Reading

The Complete Medicinal Herbal by Penelope Ody
The New Age Herbalist by Richard Mabey
The Herb Bible by Dr. Earl Mindell
The Vitamin Bible by Dr. Earl Mindell
Prescription for Nutritional Healing by James and Phyllis Balch

Resources

Herb, Vitamin & Mineral Product Manufacturers

Pharmavite
15451 San Fernando Mission Blvd
Mission Hills CA 91345
1–800–255–9811

Associations, Educational Institutes & Magazines

American Association of Naturopathic Physicans
601 Valley Street, Suite # 105
Seattle WA 98109
206–298–0125 (referrals)

Canadian Naturopathic Association
4174 Dundas Street West, # 304
Etobicoke ON M8X 1X3
416–233–1043
Fax: 416–233–2924

Herb Research Foundation
1007 Pearl Street, # 200
Boulder CO 80302
303–449–2265
1–800–748–2617
Fax: 303–449–7849

Bastyr University
14500 Juanita Drive NE
Kenmore WA 98028
425–823–1300

Dominion Herbal College
7527 Kingsway
Burnaby BC V3N 3C1
604–521–5822
Fax: 604–526–1561

Wild Rose College of Natural Healing
400 – 1228 Kensington Road NW
Calgary AB T2N 4P9
403–270–0936
Fax: 403–283–0799

alive, **Canadian Journal of Health and Nutrition**
7436 Fraser Park Drive
Burnaby BC V5J 5B9
604–435–1919
Fax: 604–435–4888

HerbalGram
PO Box 144345
Austin TX 78714–4345
512–926–4900
Fax: 512–926–2345

The Herb Companion
741 Corporate Circle
Suite "H"
PO Box 16520
Golden CO 80401
970–669–7672
Fax: 303–216–9220

Index

About the Author

Victoria Hogan, MA, is an environmentalist and natural medicine activist. She writes, lectures and gives radio interviews on those subjects. She has given numerous seminars to patients of naturopaths and medical doctors to support them in healthy diets and lifestyles. She has written weekly columns on health, fitness and food, as well as many articles on the immune system, healthy diets, and other health and environmental concerns for both women's and other magazines. She is past president of EarthSave Canada, and a former director of VUNA (Vegetarian Union of North America). Victoria resides with her husband in Vancouver, BC, Canada.

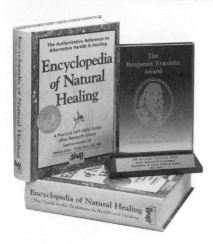
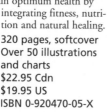
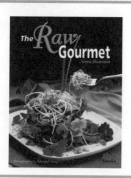

The Vegetarian Gourmet
Dagmar von Cramm

A sumptuously illustrated book featuring the best of European vegetarian cuisine.

246 pages, softcover
Over 200 full-colour photographs
$29.95 Cdn $24.95 US
ISBN 0-920470-80-7

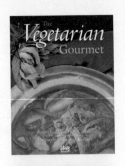

Living With Green Power
A Gourmet Collection of Living Food Recipes
Elysa Markowitz

Reap the rewards of the living foods diet, such as proper digestion, a strong immune system and an abundance of energy.

176 pages, hardcover
96 full-colour photos
$29.95 Cdn $24.95 US
ISBN 0-920470-11-4

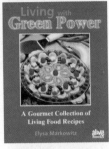

Fats that Heal, Fats that Kill
Udo Erasmus

Over 100,000 copies in print!

This book brings you the most current research on the common and less well-known oils and their therapeutic potential. *"A welcome relief from the one-sided approach of our current health authorities, who espouse the low-fat diet as the panacea for all health problems. The informed and balanced presentation will help to take the fear out of fats."* – Richard A. Kuin, MD, President of the International Society for Orthomolecular Medicine

456 pages, softcover
$27.95 Cdn $22.95 US
ISBN 0-920470-38-6

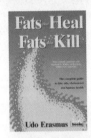

The Natural Physician
Your Health Guide for Common Ailments
Mark Stengler, ND

A straight-forward and practical guide for those who prefer to heal themselves with naturopathic medicine, herbs, vitamins, minerals and other natural remedies.

218 pages, softcover
$15.95 Cdn $12.95 US
ISBN 0-920470-46-7

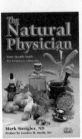

The Cultured Cabbage
Klaus Kaufmann and Annelies Schöneck

Lovers of sauerkraut and pickled vegetables will welcome this guide to the remarkable heath-enhancing properties of lactic acid-fermented foods.

80 pages, softcover
8 full-colour photographs
$11.95 Cdn $10.95 US
ISBN 0-920470-66-1

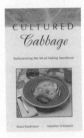
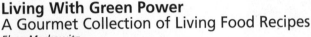

Kefir Rediscovered!
Klaus Kaufmann

The nutritional benefits of this ancient healing food are explored. Includes recipes for kefir skin-care products and kefir foods.

96 pages, softcover
$11.95 Cdn $10.95 US
ISBN 0-920470-65-3

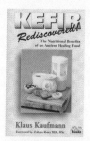

Silica
The Amazing Gel
Klaus Kaufmann

An in-depth exploration of the beneficial effects of silica gel on cancer, diabetes, gastritis, ulcers, skin disorders and teeth.

208 pages, softcover
$12.95 Cdn $9.95 US
ISBN 0-920470-30-0

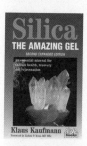

Kombucha Rediscovered!
Klaus Kaufmann

Everything you ever wanted to know about the amazing healing properties of the fermented kombucha mushroom.

96 pages, softcover
6 full-colour photographs
$11.95 Cdn $10.95 US
ISBN 0-920470-64-5

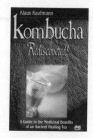

For the Love of Food
The Complete Natural Foods Cookbook
Jeanne Marie Martin

In this updated version of Martin's classic book, you'll find comprehensive guidelines for food combining, vegetarianism, fasting, vitamins and minerals, bread making, sprouting and cooking with herbs.

384 pages, hardcover
13 full-colour photographs
$29.95 Cdn $24.95 US
ISBN 0-920470-71-8

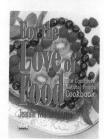

Healing with Herbal Juices
Siegfried Gursche MH

The first book of its kind, *Healing with Herbal Juices* presents a simple, effective way to benefit from the superior healing power of herbs.

156 pages, softcover
$18.95 Cdn $16.95 US
ISBN 0-920470-34-3

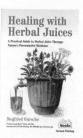

A Diet for All Reasons

Paulette Eisen

More than a cookbook, *A Diet for All Reasons* explains why a meat-, egg- and dairy-free diet is essential for cardiovascular health, reduced stress levels, and overall well-being.

176 pages, spiral bound
$15.95 Cdn $12.95 US
ISBN 0-920470-68-8

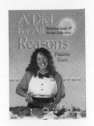

Devil's Claw Root and Other Natural Remedies for Arthritis

Rachel Carston
(updated and revised by Klaus Kaufmann)

The symptoms of arthritis can often be completely eliminated by taking devil's claw root. Find out how in this down-to earth guide.

112 pages, softcover
$11.95 Cdn $9.95 US
ISBN 0-920470-36-X

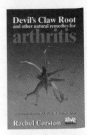

Menopause
Time for a Change

Merri Lu Park

An in-depth and practical guide that will put you in control of your life and your health.

304 pages, softcover
$18.95 Cdn $16.95 US
ISBN 0-920470-33-5

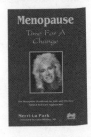

The Breuss Cancer Cure

Rudolph Breuss

The renowned Dr Breuss offers practical advice for the prevention and natural treatment of cancer, leukemia and other seemingly incurable diseases.

112 pages, softcover
$13.95 Cdn $11.95 US
ISBN 0-920470-56-4

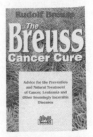

Allergies
Disease in Disguise

Dr Carolee Bateson-Koch

This is the first book to explain how to achieve complete and permanent recovery from your allergies.

224 pages, softcover
$17.95 Cdn $15.95 US
ISBN 0-920470-42-4

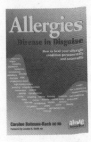

 alive books are available at health food stores and book stores or by calling 1-800-663-6513.